GI AND LIVER DISEASE DURING PREGNANCY

A Practical Approach

GI AND LIVER DISEASE DURING PREGNANCY
A Practical Approach

Edited by:

KIM L. ISAACS, MD, PHD
Professor of Medicine
University of North Carolina at Chapel Hill
Division of Gastroenterology and Hepatology
Chapel Hill, North Carolina

MILLIE D. LONG, MD, MPH
Assistant Professor of Medicine
University of North Carolina at Chapel Hill
Division of Gastroenterology and Hepatology
Chapel Hill, North Carolina

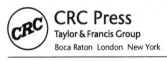

CRC Press
Taylor & Francis Group
Boca Raton London New York

CRC Press is an imprint of the
Taylor & Francis Group, an **informa** business

First published 2013 by SLACK Incorporated

Published 2024 by CRC Press
2385 NW Executive Center Drive, Suite 320, Boca Raton FL 33431

and by CRC Press
4 Park Square, Milton Park, Abingdon, Oxon, OX14 4RN

CRC Press is an imprint of Taylor & Francis Group, LLC

Library of Congress Cataloging-in-Publication Data

GI and liver disease during pregnancy : a practical approach / [edited by] Kim L. Isaacs, Millie D. Long.
    p. ; cm.
Includes bibliographical references and index.
ISBN 978-1-61711-023-8 (alk. paper)
I. Isaacs, Kim L., II. Long, Millie D.
[DNLM: 1. Gastrointestinal Diseases. 2. Pregnancy Complications. 3. Liver Diseases. WQ 240]

 618.3'64--dc23

                                        2012026369

ISBN: 9781617110238 (pbk)
ISBN: 9781003524359 (ebk)

DOI: 10.1201/9781003524359

DEDICATION

I would like to dedicate this book to my family: Steve, Ben, and Abby, who have supported me during my career in every way imaginable.

Kim L. Isaacs, MD, PhD

I would like to dedicate this book to my family: Sid, Connor, Tyler, and Helen, who are the most important influences in my life.

Millie D. Long, MD, MPH

CONTENTS

Dedication .... *v*
Acknowledgments .... *ix*
About the Editors .... *xi*
Contributing Authors .... *xiii*
Preface .... *xvii*
Foreword by Sunanda Kane, MD, MSPH .... *xix*
Introduction .... *xxi*

Chapter 1   Gastroesophageal Reflux Disease in Pregnancy 1
             Ryan D. Madanick, MD

Chapter 2   Nausea and Vomiting of Pregnancy 13
             Laurie-Anne C. Swaby, MD and Kim L. Isaacs, MD, PhD

Chapter 3   Gastric Bypass and Pregnancy 31
             D. Wayne Overby, MD

Chapter 4   Abdominal Pain in Pregnancy: Differential Diagnosis
             and Initial Work-Up of Abdominal Pain 39
             Millie D. Long, MD, MPH

Chapter 5   Constipation in Pregnancy 61
             *Yolanda V. Scarlett, MD; Kim L. Isaacs, MD, PhD; and
             Millie D. Long, MD, MPH*

Chapter 6   Irritable Bowel Syndrome 75
             Millie D. Long, MD, MPH and Spencer D. Dorn, MD, MPH

Chapter 7   Inflammatory Bowel Disease 91
             Lindsay E. Jones, MD and Millie D. Long, MD, MPH

Chapter 8   Endoscopy 117
             Kim L. Isaacs, MD, PhD

Chapter 9   Surgical Management of the Pregnant Patient ... 133
             Megan Quintana, MD and Reza Rahbar, MD

Chapter 10   Pancreatitis and Biliary Issues 153
             Patricia D. Jones, MD and Lisa M. Gangarosa, MD

Chapter 11   Chronic Liver Disease 167
             Caitlyn M. Patrick, MD and A. Sidney Barritt IV, MD, MSCR

Chapter 12   Acute Liver Disease 185
             Eric S. Orman, MD and A. Sidney Barritt IV, MD, MSCR

Appendix: Classification of Medications During Pregnancy *211*
Financial Disclosures *217*
Index *219*

ACKNOWLEDGMENTS

We would like to acknowledge all of our pregnant patients who have taught us about gastrointestinal and liver disease during pregnancy.

ABOUT THE EDITORS

Kim L. Isaacs, MD, PhD received her PhD and MD at the State University of New York at Stony Brook in 1981 and 1984, respectively. She completed her internal medicine residency and gastroenterology fellowship at the University of North Carolina at Chapel Hill in 1987 and 1991. She has been on the faculty at the University of North Carolina at Chapel Hill in the division of gastroenterology and hepatology since 1991, and is currently a professor and co-director of the University of North Carolina Inflammatory Bowel Disease Center.

Millie D. Long, MD, MPH earned her doctor of medicine degree at the University of Virginia, where she was a Bowman Scholar. She completed a residency and chief residency in internal medicine at the University of Alabama at Birmingham, and then completed a gastroenterology fellowship at the University of North Carolina at Chapel Hill. While at the University of North Carolina, she also completed a fellowship in preventive medicine, and a masters of public health in epidemiology at the Gillings School of Public Health. She is board certified in internal medicine, preventive medicine, and gastroenterology. She is currently an Assistant Professor of Medicine in the Department of Medicine. Her clinical practice is based at the University of North Carolina Inflammatory Bowel Disease Center.

Dr. Long's interests include research on prevention of complications of inflammatory bowel disease, women's health, and teaching clinical epidemiology. Dr. Long has contributed numerous peer-reviewed publications, book chapters, and review articles to medical literature. Dr. Long is a member of the American College of Gastroenterology, where she serves on the Research Committee. She is also a member of the American Gastroenterological Association and the Crohn's and Colitis Foundation of America, where she serves on the Professional Education Committee.

CONTRIBUTING AUTHORS

A. Sidney Barritt IV, MD, MSCR (Chapters 11 and 12)
Assistant Professor of Medicine
University of North Carolina at Chapel Hill
Division of Gastroenterology and Hepatology
Chapel Hill, North Carolina

Spencer D. Dorn, MD, MPH (Chapter 6)
Assistant Professor of Medicine
University of North Carolina at Chapel Hill
Division of Gastroenterology and Hepatology
Chapel Hill, North Carolina

Lisa M. Gangarosa, MD (Chapter 10)
Clinical Professor of Medicine
University of North Carolina at Chapel Hill
Division of Gastroenterology and Hepatology
Chapel Hill, North Carolina

Sunanda Kane, MD, MSPH (Foreword)
Miles and Shirley Fitterman Division of Gastroenterology and
Hepatology
Mayo Clinic College of Medicine
Rochester, Minnesota

Lindsay E. Jones, MD (Chapter 7)
Division of Gastroenterology
Walter Reed National Military Medical Center
Department of Medicine
Bethesda, Maryland

Patricia D. Jones, MD (Chapter 10)
Fellow in Gastroenterology and Hepatology
University of North Carolina at Chapel Hill
Chapel Hill, North Carolina

Ryan D. Madanick, MD (Chapter 1)
Assistant Professor of Medicine
Director, UNC Gastroenterology and Hepatology Fellowship Program
University of North Carolina School of Medicine
Division of Gastroenterology and Hepatology
Center for Esophageal Diseases and Swallowing
Chapel Hill, North Carolina

Eric S. Orman, MD (Chapter 12)
Fellow in Transplant Hepatology
University of North Carolina
Division of Gastroenterology and Hepatology
Chapel Hill, North Carolina

D. Wayne Overby, MD (Chapter 3)
Assistant Professor of Surgery
University of North Carolina at Chapel Hill
Division of Gastrointestinal Surgery
Chapel Hill, North Carolina

Caitlyn M. Patrick, MD (Chapter 11)
Resident Physician
University of North Carolina
Department of Internal Medicine
Chapel Hill, North Carolina

Megan Quintana, MD (Chapter 9)
Surgical Resident
University of North Carolina at Chapel Hill
Department of Surgery
Chapel Hill, North Carolina

Reza Rahbar, MD (Chapter 9)
Assistant Professor of Surgery
University of North Carolina at Chapel Hill
Division of Gastrointestinal Surgery
Chapel Hill, North Carolina

Yolanda V. Scarlett, MD (Chapter 5)
Associate Professor of Medicine
University of North Carolina at Chapel Hill
Division of Gastroenterology and Hepatology
Chapel Hill, North Carolina

Laurie-Anne C. Swaby, MD (Chapter 2)
Fellow in Gastroenterology and Hepatology
University of North Carolina at Chapel Hill
Chapel Hill, North Carolina

PREFACE

As female gastroenterologists, we are often sent female patients, both out of patient choice and physician choice. This is especially true for the pregnant patient with gastrointestinal illness. Pregnancy and pregnant patients tend to cause anxiety in physicians who do not care for them on a routine basis due to concerns about the effects of evaluation and management on the new life. Too often the impulse is to wait until pregnancy is complete before dealing with medical issues that arise. We both have also had patients with inflammatory bowel disease who, once pregnant, were told by well-meaning physicians to stop all of their medications so that there would be no injury to the fetus. Many of these women then had a flare of their disease activity and a miserable pregnancy. We wrote this book to help our patients so they could receive good care, taking into account the effects on the growing fetus. We also wrote this book for practicing physicians (gastroenterologists, surgeons, and obstetricians) to review the management of gastrointestinal illness as it applies to the pregnant patient and to decrease the anxiety that arises when approaching a pregnant patient. We wanted to make this a practitioner-friendly handbook that could be a ready reference in the clinic, hospital, and endoscopy suite. We have both been involved in the day-to-day care of pregnant patients with inflammatory bowel disease and have coauthors that have expertise in other areas of gastroenterology. We hope that you will find this handbook format helpful in evaluating and managing gastrointestinal illness in the pregnant patient.

Kim Isaacs, MD, PhD
Millie Long, MD, MPH
University of North Carolina at Chapel Hill
July 6, 2012

FOREWORD

Nothing strikes fear into a gastroenterologist more than a patient referred with gastrointestinal symptoms during pregnancy. Sources for information come from UpToDate, colleagues, and key opinion leaders. But who has time to make a call and play phone tag, hunt down a colleague rounding in the hospital, or sit at a computer and read? Finally, there is now a handy resource that readily fits into a pocket or on your bookshelf for those instances where you need to consider a broad range of conditions. *GI and Liver Disease During Pregnancy: A Practical Approach* is aptly named. Twelve chapters divided into complaints or discrete diseases make it easy to find what you are looking for. Each chapter covers epidemiology, pathology, presentation, management, and a summary. After each section are key points in a highlighted box, exactly what a busy clinician needs. In addition, there are tables with medications and their FDA category, which would really come in handy at the bedside or in the office. "Alternative" therapies are listed as well. The references are current and the authors truly provide hands-on practical recommendations. It was easy to read, I finished it cover to cover in under 2 hours. A chapter that I appreciate and would not have thought to include just 5 years ago was care in a patient status postbariatric surgery. Thank you Drs. Isaacs and Long for providing the GI community with such a valuable and useable reference. Did I mention that this would be a great resource for Board review as well?

Sunanda Kane, MD, MSPH
Miles and Shirley Fitterman Division of Gastroenterology and Hepatology
Mayo Clinic College of Medicine
Rochester, Minnesota

INTRODUCTION

As female gastroenterologists, we are often asked to consult in cases where pregnant women have ongoing gastrointestinal symptoms. We discovered a lack of readily available resources regarding how to work-up and manage these symptoms in pregnant women. Therefore, this practical handbook on gastrointestinal disorders in pregnancy was born.

The book is arranged in 12 individual chapters focusing on common gastrointestinal ailments and conditions during pregnancy. The topics were selected based on clinical scenarios that we commonly see in our practices. For example, there is a chapter on constipation and hemorrhoids, both of which are seen frequently in pregnant women. However, there are also chapters dealing with chronic gastrointestinal conditions that require in-depth, ongoing medical and nutritional management during pregnancy. We have included chapters on chronic liver diseases, inflammatory bowel diseases, and even on women who have undergone prior gastric bypass. Due to these gastrointestinal conditions, these women often require special consideration and management during pregnancy. We have also included chapters meant to help with the diagnostic work-up of pregnant women with gastrointestinal symptoms. There is a chapter detailing the differential diagnosis and work-up of abdominal pain during pregnancy. There is also a chapter on the surgical management of various disorders during pregnancy, such as appendicitis or acute cholecystitis. We feel that this series of concise chapters will aid providers in caring for pregnant women with gastrointestinal symptoms and disorders.

The layout of the book is meant to be user-friendly. Each chapter focuses on the epidemiology, pathophysiology, diagnostic work-up, and treatment of the gastrointestinal condition. There are highlighted key points throughout each chapter that can be used for quick reference or bedside counseling of the pregnant patient. Importantly, in each chapter there is a medication and breastfeeding guide to allow effective counseling on the safety of various medications. These guides were written with the current pregnancy grading system in mind, as many providers are familiar with this A, B, C, D, X guidance system. An appendix details changes to the grading system that will be implemented over the next several years.

We hope that you will find this practical handbook useful in your clinical practice. We wrote this book with you, the busy provider, in mind. We enjoyed working with our colleagues who contributed outstanding chapters to this book. Most importantly, we hope that this practical guide will aid you in your care of pregnant women with gastrointestinal disorders.

1

Gastroesophageal Reflux Disease in Pregnancy

Ryan D. Madanick, MD

INTRODUCTION AND EPIDEMIOLOGY

Heartburn, or pyrosis, is the cardinal symptom of gastroesophageal reflux disease (GERD) and occurs in up to 80% of women during pregnancy.[1] Heartburn can occur during any trimester of the pregnancy. The onset of heartburn in pregnancy occurs in the first trimester in 22% to 52% of women, and the prevalence of heartburn increases with gestational age.[2,3] Atypical symptoms of GERD such as cough, chest pain, and globus also occur with higher frequency than in the prepregnancy state.[4] Because of the high prevalence of heartburn and GERD in pregnant women, special consideration should be given to the pathophysiology and management of heartburn and GERD during pregnancy.

Isaacs KL, Long MD.
*GI and Liver Disease During Pregnancy:
A Practical Approach (pp. 1-12).*
© 2013 Taylor & Francis Group

KEY POINTS

- Heartburn occurs in 80% of women during pregnancy.
- It can occur in any trimester.
- It increases with gestational age.
- Atypical symptoms are common (cough, chest pain, globus).

PATHOPHYSIOLOGY

In nonpregnant patients, several physiologic abnormalities work together to lead to GERD, including a defective antireflux barrier, the lower esophageal sphincter (LES), impaired esophageal clearance of refluxate, and an altered mucosal barrier.[5] During pregnancy, increased intra-abdominal pressure from an enlarging, gravid uterus may lead to an increase in reflux, but this anatomic change does not explain the onset of symptoms in early pregnancy. In asymptomatic pregnant women, mean LES pressure is lower than in nonpregnant women even before the 20th week of pregnancy, despite the same intra-abdominal pressure.[6] However, in pregnant women with heartburn, resting LES pressure decreases progressively through gestation more often than those without heartburn and returns to normal pressure after delivery.[7] These alterations in LES function appear to result from changes in the hormonal milieu during pregnancy.[8,9]

KEY POINTS

- LES pressure is lower in pregnancy.
- LES pressure decreases progressively through gestation.

PRESENTATION AND EVALUATION

The diagnosis of GERD in pregnant women occurs in much the same way as in nonpregnant patients. The cardinal symptom of GERD is heartburn, or pyrosis, a retrosternal burning sensation that radiates upward from the epigastrium toward the neck. Patients with new-onset heartburn can be presumptively diagnosed with GERD related to pregnancy and treated appropriately (see Management). Additional studies should be limited to reduce the potential for harm to the fetus. Barium radiographs should be avoided. Esophageal manometry and reflux testing (with pH only or combined pH-impedance testing) are rarely indicated during pregnancy, although they may be performed safely if necessary.[10] Endoscopy should be limited to pregnant women with severe, refractory symptoms or complicated GERD.

KEY POINTS
• Clinical diagnosis is based on symptoms.
• Testing, such as endoscopy, should be limited only to women with severe, refractory symptoms.

MANAGEMENT

The safety of medical therapy during pregnancy is shown in Table 1-1.

ANTACIDS

Antacids have no FDA pregnancy classification. Calcium-, magnesium-, and aluminum-based antacids have not had teratogenic effects in animal studies. These antacids are believed to be safe for human use during pregnancy in standard doses, although each antacid has theoretical risks to the fetus.[11,12] In supratherapeutic doses, calcium-based antacids (eg, calcium carbonate) can result in milk-alkali syndrome, characterized by the triad of hypercalcemia, metabolic alkalosis, and renal insufficiency.[13,14] Theoretically, high doses of aluminum-containing antacids could cause fetal neurotoxicity, and magnesium-containing antacids could lead to tocolysis. Antacids with sodium bicarbonate are not safe during pregnancy because of the risk for maternal or fetal metabolic alkalosis and fluid overload. Magnesium trisilicate, a component of antacids such as Gaviscon (Reckitt Benckiser, Inc, Slough, UK), can induce fetal nephrolithiasis, hypotonia, respiratory distress, and cardiovascular impairment in long-term or high-dose use.

Table 1-1

Medications for Use in the Treatment of Heartburn and Gastroesophageal Reflux Disease

Drug	FDA Pregnancy Category*	Pregnancy Comment	Breastfeeding Comment
Antacids			
Aluminum containing	None	Most low risk: minimal absorption	Low risk
Calcium containing	None	Most low risk: minimal absorption	Low risk
Magnesium containing	None	Most low risk: minimal absorption	Low risk
Magnesium trisilicates	None	Avoid long-term or high doses	Low risk
Sodium bicarbonate	None	Not safe: alkalosis	Low risk
Mucosal Protectants			
Sucralfate	B	Low risk	No human data: probably compatible
H2-Receptor Antagonists			
Cimetidine	B	Controlled data: low risk	Compatible
Famotidine	B	Paucity of safety data	Limited human data: probably compatible
Nizatidine	B	Limited human data: low risk in animals	Limited human data: probably compatible
Ranitidine	B	Low risk	Limited human data: probably compatible

(continued)

Table 1-1 *(continued)*

Medications for Use in the Treatment of Heartburn and Gastroesophageal Reflux Disease

Drug	FDA Pregnancy Category*	Pregnancy Comment	Breastfeeding Comment
Proton Pump Inhibitors			
Esomeprazole	B	Limited data: low risk	No human data: potential toxicity
Lansoprazole	B	Limited data: low risk	No human data: potential toxicity
Omeprazole	C	Embryonic and fetal toxicity reported, but large data sets suggest low risk	Limited human data: potential toxicity
Pantoprazole	B	Limited data: low risk	No human data: potential toxicity
Rabeprazole	B	Limited data: low risk	No human data: potential toxicity
Promotility Agents			
Cisapride	C	Controlled study: low risk, limited availability	Limited human data: probably compatible
Metoclopramide	B	Low risk	Limited human data: potential toxicity

Adapted from Mahadevan U, Kane S. American Gastroenterological Association Institute medical position statement on the use of gastrointestinal medications in pregnancy. *Gastroenterology.* 2006;131(1):278-282.

*See appendix for discussion of FDA pregnancy categories.

HISTAMINE-2-RECEPTOR ANTAGONISTS

All histamine-2-receptor antagonists (H2RAs) are FDA Pregnancy Category B.[11] In a meta-analysis of 4 cohort studies comprising 2398 exposed and 119,892 unexposed subjects, the overall odds ratio for congenital malformations after in utero exposure to H2RAs was not statistically significant.[15] Likewise, the incidence of spontaneous abortions, preterm delivery, and being small for gestational age was not a significant statistical difference between exposed and unexposed groups.

Among individual H2RAs, cimetidine and ranitidine have the largest amount of data to support their safety. Famotidine and nizatidine have limited data that neither confirms or refutes their safety. Cimetidine has a weak antiandrogenic effect in animal studies, but sexual defects have not been reported in humans.[16]

PROTON PUMP INHIBITORS

All proton pump inhibitors (PPIs) are FDA Pregnancy Category B, except omeprazole, which is Category C.[11] In a meta-analysis of 7 cohort studies that included 1530 PPI-exposed pregnancies, newborns exposed to PPI during pregnancy did not demonstrate a statistically significant rate of major fetal malformations compared with newborns who were not exposed to PPI.[17]

In a subsequent large Danish cohort study of 840,968 live births, the prevalence of major congenital defects was 3.4% among infants whose mothers were exposed to PPIs during either the first trimester or during the 4-week period prior to pregnancy compared with 2.6% among those who were not exposed (adjusted odds ratio [AOR] 1.23; 95% CI, 1.05 to 1.44).[18] However, the increased prevalence of birth defects only occurred among infants whose mothers had received PPI therapy during the 4 weeks prior to conception (AOR 1.39; 95% CI, 1.10 to 1.76) but not among the group exposed only during first trimester (AOR 1.10; 95% CI, 0.91 to 1.34). None of the individual PPIs was associated with an increased prevalence of birth defects. Lansoprazole was the only PPI for which use during the preconception period was associated with a statistically significant risk, although limited data were available for rabeprazole. Dexlansoprazole was not included in this analysis.

OTHER AGENTS

The promotility agent metoclopramide is a Category B drug.[11] Although its principal use during pregnancy is for nausea and vomiting of pregnancy, metoclopramide can increase LES tone, esophageal acid clearance, and gastric emptying.[1] In a study of 113,612 singleton births, exposure to metoclopramide during the first trimester was not associated with an increased odds of major congenital malformations or adverse fetal outcomes when compared with nonexposure to the drug.[19]

Sucralfate is Pregnancy Category B.[11] Sucralfate inhibits pepsin activity and protects the gastrointestinal mucosa. The major risk of sucralfate relates to its aluminum content, but an increased risk for adverse fetal outcomes has not been observed.

Selecting Therapy for a Pregnant Woman

Because the teratogenic potential of any medication is a major concern in pregnant women, women should limit pharmacotherapy until after the critical period of organogenesis, which ends after the 10th week of gestation. Although most acid-reducing medications are considered safe for use during pregnancy, none is completely without risk to the fetus. Patients should be informed of the available data, as well as the possibility that unknown fetal risks could still remain.

If possible, the first line of therapy should be lifestyle and dietary changes (Table 1-2) for women with new-onset heartburn. Lifestyle modifications include avoidance of alcohol, tobacco, and refluxogenic medications. Women should limit their intake of foods that can induce heartburn and reflux, such as chocolate, peppermint, and citrus products, and should eat small, frequent (every 2 to 3 hours), low-fat meals. The addition of chewing gum between meals can help stimulate salivary secretions, which alkalinizes the esophageal lumen and reduces esophageal acid exposure (avoid mint-flavored chewing gum). Patients with nocturnal heartburn or regurgitation should elevate the head of the bed by 6 inches and avoid eating within 3 hours of reclining. Basic lifestyle modifications can resolve symptoms in up to 25% of patients.[5]

If lifestyle changes do not adequately reduce symptoms in pregnant women with heartburn, a step-up approach to pharmacotherapy is advocated. Antacids are the first line of medical therapy for symptom relief. An antacid chewing gum containing calcium

Table 1-2

Lifestyle Modifications in the Treatment of Heartburn and Gastroesophageal Reflux Disease

- Elevation of head of the bed
- Dietary modifications
    - ∞ Low-fat, high-protein diet
    - ∞ Fast for 2 to 3 hours before sleeping
    - ∞ Avoid specific irritants (citrus juices, tomato products, peppermint, coffee, alcohol)
    - ∞ Avoid chocolate
- Stop smoking
- Avoid GERD-provocative medications
    - ∞ Anticholinergics
    - ∞ Sedatives/tranquilizers
    - ∞ Theophylline
    - ∞ Prostaglandins
    - ∞ Calcium channel blockers

carbonate (CHOOZ [Insight Pharmaceuticals Corp, Langhorn, PA]) is available commercially and can provide patients with a portable, on-demand option. If symptoms do not respond to antacids, patients should start an H2RA. Twice-daily dosing of the H2RA is more likely to achieve symptomatic response than once-daily dosing.[20] Should symptoms continue despite H2RAs, PPIs should be used. The key limitation of both the H2RAs and the PPIs is their onset of action, which is not rapid enough for immediate symptom relief.

When a woman has already been using a PPI prior to pregnancy, physicians should discuss the indications for the PPI compared with the teratogenic potential as early as possible so that she can make an informed decision. Women should remain on a PPI if they are known to have significant complications of GERD, such as Barrett's esophagus or a severe peptic stricture. Women without complicated GERD should attempt to step down their PPI dose if possible, especially during the first trimester. Some women may be able to step down to an H2RA or even antacids if their symptoms remain tolerable. Although PPI exposure during the first trimester appears to be safe, most authorities would recommend discontinuing the drug at least through the first trimester if possible.

Preconception Counseling

With women of childbearing age who are taking medications for GERD prior to pregnancy, physicians should review the indications for the medications and the possible teratogenic risks prior to any planned pregnancy. Women with complicated disease should be advised to remain on their chronic medical therapy. Although use of PPIs is generally considered safe during pregnancy, PPI use in the 4 weeks prior to conception could slightly increase the risk of birth defects.[18] Therefore, women without known complications should attempt to step down therapy to an H2RA or antacids if possible, at least through conception and the first trimester.

Medical Therapy During Lactation

Most women who develop heartburn during pregnancy will experience relief of their symptoms following delivery. However, some women will have persistent symptoms or will require therapy for complicated GERD. Antacids are considered to be safe during lactation. All H2RAs and PPIs are excreted in breast milk, but limited data are available to guide use and safety of these during lactation. H2RAs are considered to be safe for use during lactation. Famotidine is the least concentrated in breast milk.[12] Because of the paucity of data, PPIs are not recommended during lactation, even though toxicity and negative outcomes have not been demonstrated.[11]

SUMMARY

Heartburn affects a majority of pregnant women at some point during gestation. In pregnant women without evidence of complicated GERD, therapy can be started without initiating a significant workup. As data continue to accumulate, medical therapy with H2RAs and PPIs during pregnancy appears to show a low risk for serious birth defects. Nonetheless, although medical therapy for GERD is generally safe during pregnancy, physicians and pregnant women need to balance the benefits of therapy with the teratogenic potential of medications.

REFERENCES

1. Richter JE. Review article: the management of heartburn in pregnancy. *Aliment Pharmacol Ther.* 2005;22(9):749-757.

2. Castro LP. Reflux esophagitis as the cause of heartburn in pregnancy. *Am J Obstet Gynecol.* 1967;98(1):1-10.

3. Marrero JM, Goggin PM, de Caestecker JS, Pearce JM, Maxwell JD. Determinants of pregnancy heartburn. *Br J Obstet Gynaecol.* 1992;99(9):731-734.

4. Rey E, Rodriguez-Artalejo F, Herraiz MA, et al. Atypical symptoms of gastro-esophageal reflux during pregnancy. *Rev Esp Enferm Dig.* 2011;103(3): 129-132.

5. Katz PO, Castell DO. Gastroesophageal reflux disease during pregnancy. *Gastroenterol Clin North Am.* 1998;27(1):153-167.

6. Bainbridge ET, Temple JG, Nicholas SP, Newton JR, Boriah V. Symptomatic gastro-esophageal reflux in pregnancy: a comparative study of white Europeans and Asians in Birmingham. *Br J Clin Pract.* 1983;37(2):53-57.

7. Nagler R, Spiro HM. Heartburn in late pregnancy: manometric studies of esophageal motor function. *J Clin Invest.* 1961;40:954-970.

8. Van Thiel DH, Gavaler JS, Stremple J. Lower esophageal sphincter pressure in women using sequential oral contraceptives. *Gastroenterology.* 1976;71(2): 232-234.

9. Schulze K, Christensen J. Lower sphincter of the opossum esophagus in pseudopregnancy. *Gastroenterology.* 1977;73(5):1082-1085.

10. Al-Amri SM. Twenty-four hour pH monitoring during pregnancy and at postpartum: a preliminary study. *Eur J Obstet Gynecol Reprod Biol.* 2002;102(2): 127-130.

11. Mahadevan U, Kane S. American Gastroenterological Association Institute technical review on the use of gastrointestinal medications in pregnancy. *Gastroenterology.* 2006;131(1):283-311.

12. Mahadevan U. Gastrointestinal medications in pregnancy. *Best Pract Res Clin Gastroenterol.* 2007;21(5):849-877.

13. Morton A. Milk-alkali syndrome in pregnancy, associated with elevated levels of parathyroid hormone-related protein. *Intern Med J.* 2002;32(9-10):492-493.

14. Gordon MV, McMahon LP, Hamblin PS. Life-threatening milk-alkali syndrome resulting from antacid ingestion during pregnancy. *Med J Aust.* 2005;182(7):350-351.

15. Gill SK, O'Brien L, Koren G. The safety of histamine 2 (H2) blockers in pregnancy: a meta-analysis. *Dig Dis Sci.* 2009;54(9):1835-1838.

16. Richter JE. Gastroesophageal reflux disease during pregnancy. *Gastroenterol Clin North Am.* 2003;32(1):235-261.

17. Gill SK, O'Brien L, Einarson TR, Koren G. The safety of proton pump inhibitors (PPIs) in pregnancy: a meta-analysis. *Am J Gastroenterol.* 2009;104(6): 1541-1545.

18. Pasternak B, Hviid A. Use of proton-pump inhibitors in early pregnancy and the risk of birth defects. *N Engl J Med.* 2010;363(22):2114-2123.

19. Matok I, Gorodischer R, Koren G, et al. The safety of metoclopramide use in the first trimester of pregnancy. *N Engl J Med.* 2009;360(24):2528-2535.

20. Larson JD, Patatanian E, Miner PB Jr, Rayburn WF, Robinson MG. Double-blind, placebo-controlled study of ranitidine for gastroesophageal reflux symptoms during pregnancy. *Obstet Gynecol.* 1997;90(1):83-87.

2

Nausea and Vomiting of Pregnancy

Laurie-Anne C. Swaby, MD and Kim L. Isaacs, MD, PhD

Nausea and vomiting of pregnancy (NVP) is common and can affect up to 50% to 90% of pregnancies with an increased likelihood of recurrence in subsequent pregnancies. Though traditionally termed *morning sickness*, most women experience NVP throughout the day with only 2% exhibiting symptoms isolated to the morning.[1] Symptoms are usually mild and limited to the first trimester with resolution by 20 weeks gestational age; however, severe refractory symptoms or hyperemesis gravidarum (HG) can occur in up to 2% of pregnancies and may cause significant morbidity to both mother and fetus. In addition to the possibility of intrauterine growth retardation (IUGR) or preterm labor as a consequence of severe symptoms, those with even mild to moderate symptoms may report significant psychosocial distress from disruption of daily activities, inability to complete social and professional responsibilities, or strain to interpersonal relationships. Even with mild to moderate symptoms, up to 20% of women experiencing NVP may use pharmacologic therapy.[2] Given the potential medical and psychosocial impacts of NVP on both mother and fetus, recognition and treatment of NVP is important. Equally important is the ability to

Isaacs KL, Long MD.
*GI and Liver Disease During Pregnancy:
A Practical Approach (pp. 13-30).*
© 2013 Taylor & Francis Group

differentiate NVP from other etiologies of these symptoms that would require alternative therapies.

EPIDEMIOLOGY

Nausea and vomiting usually present between the 4th and 6th week of gestation and peak between the 8th and 12th weeks. The development of nausea and/or emesis after 20 weeks gestational age should raise the suspicion for other etiologies. NVP is more common in younger women, primigravidas, obese women, multiparous pregnancies, nonsmokers, and those with a lower educational level.[3]

KEY POINTS
• For nausea and vomiting after 20 weeks gestational age, think about other etiologies.   • NVP is usually mild with resolution by 20 weeks gestational age.   • Two percent of women experience severe disabling symptoms with increased maternal and fetal morbidity.

PATHOPHYSIOLOGY

The pathophysiology of NVP is not well understood; however, there are multiple theories invoking hormonal variations, fetal protection, evolution, vestibular effects, gastrointestinal distress, hyperolfaction, psychological factors, and genetics.

METABOLIC AND HORMONAL FACTORS

The peak incidence of NVP correlates with peak levels of human chorionic gonadotropin (hCG) at 12 to 14 weeks gestational age. This association has been supported by the increased severity of symptoms in conditions with higher hCG levels, such as molar pregnancies, multiple gestations, and Trisomy 21 (Downs syndrome), but remains controversial as some women continue to vomit even later in pregnancy when hCG levels fall.[4]

Elevated levels of estrogen and progesterone lead to an increased production of nitric oxide, which promotes relaxation of smooth muscle, thereby slowing gastrointestinal (GI) motility and causing relative gastroparesis. Hyperthyroidism is a rare cause of NVP.[5] Immune system dysregulation in the setting of increased fetal cell-free DNA, promotion of maternal immunogenicity and trophoblast damage, as well as predominance of Th1 cells and the release of inflammatory cytokines may also play a role in the development of NVP.[6]

GASTROINTESTINAL MOTILITY

In addition to the hormone-induced reduction of gastric motility outlined above, alterations in lower esophageal sphincter pressure and resultant gastroesophageal reflux may manifest with nausea and contribute to NVP. Progressive uterine enlargement contributes to decreased gastric emptying and promotion of reflux.

HELICOBACTER PYLORI

Studies suggest an increased association of *Helicobacter pylori* infection with NVP and HG. Despite this association, the vast majority of women who are currently or were previously infected with *H pylori* do not exhibit severe NVP or HG, and, therefore, universal testing of *H pylori* status is not recommended, but can be considered in refractory cases as this may decrease symptoms in select individuals.[7]

KEY POINT
• Check for *H pylori* in patients with refractory symptoms.

FETAL PROTECTION

Although severe NVP is associated with low birth weights, intrauterine growth retardation, and preterm delivery as a consequence of maternal malnutrition and fetal distress, studies show a consistent decrease in miscarriage rates in women with mild to moderate NVP with a common odds ratio of 0.36 (95% CI: 0.32 to 0.42)[8] as well as reductions in perinatal death, premature delivery, and low birth weight.[8,9] Some theorize that avoidance of certain foods as a consequence of NVP may reduce fetal exposure to potentially harmful bacteria or toxins.[10] Despite the multitude of theories, no consensus exists, as NVP may reflect a heterogeneous and complex interplay of multiple factors.

HYPEREMESIS GRAVIDARUM

HG is a more severe form of NVP, affecting between 0.5% and 3% of pregnancies. Unlike NVP, which is thought to confer a feto-protective role, HG is associated with significant maternal and fetal morbidity given the associated complications of dehydration, electrolyte imbalance, nutritional deficiency, catabolism/ketonuria, and weight loss of more than 5% of prepregnancy weight by definition. Risk factors include nulliparity, multiple gestations, trophoblastic disease, prior HG (15% recurrence risk), fetal chromosomal and/or anatomic abnormalities, family history of HG, obesity, and female fetus.[11] The proposed pathophysiology of HG overlaps with NVP with particular emphasis on the implication of altered immunogenicity to pregnancy with an exaggerated Th1 cell response, thereby inducing IL-4, TNF-alpha, and other cytokines.[12,13]

The modified Pregnancy-Unique Quantification of Emesis (PUQE) score for NVP incorporates the number of daily vomiting episodes, duration of nausea per day in hours, and the number of retching episodes with a minimum score of 3 and a maximum score of 15 (mild: <6, moderate: 7 to 12, and severe: ≥13). Though successful term pregnancies are possible with HG, the associated morbidity places considerable demand on the health care system as these patients may require multiple hospitalizations to address dehydration and nutritional deficiencies with rare complications including Mallory-Weiss tears, esophageal rupture, retinal hemorrhage, Wernicke's encephalopathy, and central pontine myelinolysis, in addition to others. Fortunately, the majority of cases of HG improve by 20 weeks gestation, but up to 10% of women may experience symptoms throughout pregnancy.[14,15]

DIFFERENTIAL DIAGNOSIS

Although most cases of NVP are benign and self-limited, the differential diagnosis of NVP is broad and includes gastroesophageal reflux, peptic ulcer disease, small-bowel obstruction, acute cholecystitis, biliary colic, pancreatitis, appendicitis, gastroenteritis, nephrolithiasis, urinary tract infection, pyelonephritis, hepatitis, complications of diabetes such as diabetic ketoacidosis (DKA), hyperthyroidism, Addison's disease, hypercalcemia, porphyria, ovarian torsion, central nervous system diseases such as migraines, labyrinthitis, Meniere's disease, vestibular dysfunction, and pre-eclampsia/hemolysis, elevated liver enzymes, and low platelet count syndrome (HELLP), acute fatty liver of pregnancy, or adverse drug effects.[16]

TESTING

In addition to a routine physical examination, the physician may consider additional diagnostic evaluation based on the individual presentation and initial assessment to exclude other etiologies of nausea and vomiting. This may include white blood cell count, serum chemistry to assess electrolytes and evaluate renal function, liver enzyme profile, amylase/lipase, thyroid panel, urinalysis, and serum glucose. Though radiographic or endoscopic studies are usually not required, upper endoscopy and abdominal ultrasound are safe in all stages of pregnancy. Although there is no known risk of magnetic resonance imaging (MRI) in pregnancy and no deleterious effects have been noted, the safety of MRI is not proven.[17,18]

KEY POINTS
• Tailor testing to differential diagnosis.
• Laboratory testing should include complete blood count (CBC), glucose, electrolytes, creatinine, liver enzyme panel, urinalysis, and thyroid panel.
• Upper endoscopy and abdominal ultrasound are safe in all pregnancy stages.

THERAPIES

NONPHARMACOLOGIC

DIETARY

Women affected by NVP and HG may decrease portion size and increase frequency of meals to maintain adequate caloric intake. In addition to avoiding personal trigger foods based on temperature, taste, or texture, affected women should avoid spicy and odiferous foods as well as those with high fat content, which may be associated with delayed gastric emptying. Additionally, recommendations for eating a small, carbohydrate-rich snack prior to rising in the morning, active hydration (>2 L/day) with separation of solid food and liquid intake, and avoidance of hunger or oversatiety have been proposed to mitigate symptoms. An increased protein content in meals may be associated with decreased incidence and severity of NVP.[19] The American College of Obstetricians and Gynecologists (ACOG) also recommends preconception multivitamins as a preventative measure; however, iron-containing vitamins may provoke nausea and may need to be held for a few weeks until symptoms abate. Altering the brand, formulation, or dosing interval (divided doses) of multivitamins may be beneficial.[20] ACOG supports the use of ginger capsules as therapy for NVP (see complementary section on p. 22).

KEY POINTS
• Eat multiple small meals.
• Eat a small, carbohydrate-rich snack prior to rising in the morning.
• Practice active hydration, >2 L/day.

LIFESTYLE CHANGES

Implementation of stress reduction techniques, including exercise, frequent naps, or decreased work requirements, has been reported to be helpful in reducing the severity of symptoms in NVP.[21]

PHARMACOLOGIC

PYRIDOXINE (VITAMIN B₆)

Pyridoxine is a water-soluble B-complex vitamin required for the metabolism of lipids, carbohydrates, and amino acids and may be administered orally in doses of 75 to 100 mg daily. Although there is no conclusive evidence of low levels of pyridoxine in patients with NVP, 2 randomized, double-blind, placebo-controlled trials support its positive impact on the reduction of the severity of nausea and the frequency of vomiting in those with moderate to severe symptoms of NVP.[22,23] Contrary to prior data, a recent study from Tan and colleagues did not show a significant benefit of the addition of pyridoxine to intravenous hydration and metoclopramide in hospitalized patients with hyperemesis gravidarum.[24]

DOXYLAMINE-PYRIDOXINE

Bendectin (doxylamine-pyridoxine) was the first drug with a specific FDA indication for NVP. Although it was voluntarily removed from the United States market due to alleged concerns for teratogenicity, further investigation did not support these claims.[25] During the time of its widespread use, rates of hospitalization for severe NVP decreased, with subsequent increase in rates postwithdrawal from the market. Doxylamine is a histamine 1-receptor blocker with proven safety and is marketed over-the-counter as Unisom SleepTabs (Chattem, Inc, Chattanooga, TN). Currently, the medication can be compounded to the recommended concentration of doxylamine 10 mg–pyridoxine 10 mg with recommended dosage of 1 to 2 tablets by mouth once or twice daily. Studies have not shown a treatment response in HG.

ANTIHISTAMINES/ANTICHOLINERGICS

Through direct antagonism of the histamine 1-receptor and consequent impact on the vestibular system and vomiting center, medications such as diphenhydramine (25 to 50 mg orally every 4 to 6 hours as needed, or 10 to 50 mg IM/IV every 4 to 6 hours as needed), meclizine (25 mg orally every 4 to 6 hours as needed), and dimenhydrinate (50 to 100 mg orally or rectally every 4 to 6 hours as needed) are used to treat NVP. With decades of research, these medications show a significant rate of efficacy with no significant risk to the fetus. Scopolamine, another anticholinergic medication, may be effective in treating NVP but is reported to cause sister-chromatid exchanges, resulting in congenital malformations. Therefore, its use in the first trimester is not recommended, and it is not considered a first-line agent.

DOPAMINE ANTAGONISTS

Medications within this class, such as prochlorperazine, promethazine, and metoclopramide, are considered second-line agents in the United States, but are widely used abroad. Through effects on the dopamine 2-receptors, they are thought to exert antiemetic effects by blocking dopamine-mediated inhibition of gastric motility as well as through actions at the chemoreceptor trigger zone.[26] The phenothiazines (prochlorperazine and promethazine) have been widely studied with no evidence of deleterious impact to the fetus. Although there was initial concern over the use of metoclopramide in the United States, it is used widely abroad, and safety data, including a population-based study in Israel from 1998 to 2007, show no increased risk to the fetus after exposure in the first trimester.[27] One prospective study from the Maternity-Pediatric Section of the French Institute of Health and Medical Research showed increased risk of fetal malformation in women taking metoclopramide (3.5% versus 1.6%); however, critics point to the lower-than-expected rate of malformations in the control group as well as the presence of potential confounders, such as alcohol intake and duration of therapy.[28] Adverse events unrelated to pregnancy, such as tardive dyskinesia, can occur but are of low frequency, prompting current recommendations to limit dosing of 10 mg orally 3 times a day for up to 3 months. A randomized controlled trial comparing the effects of promethazine 25 mg IV every 8 hours versus metoclopramide 10 mg IV every 8 hours for 24 hours in women during their first hospitalization for HG showed no difference in treatment response but showed a superior side effect profile in those receiving metoclopramide.[29] In a small sample, the use of another dopamine antagonist, droperidol, was associated with shorter hospitalizations and decreased re-admissions without negative impact on maternal-fetal outcomes.[30] Notably, droperidol bears a black-box warning for associations with QT prolongation and cardiac arrhythmias, requiring serial EKGs with administration. This has resulted in its very limited use currently.

Serotonin Antagonists

Safety data on the use of ondansetron in the treatment of nausea and vomiting of pregnancy are limited, and clear benefit over other agents, such as phenothiazines, is not yet proven. Ondansetron exerts its effects via antagonism of serotonin receptors in the small bowel and medullary vomiting center. In the small sample size from case reports and small randomized controlled trials, there does not appear to be any evidence of significant adverse fetal effects with its use. However, analysis of data from the National Birth Defects Prevention Study show a possible association between ondansetron and cleft palate (OR = 2.37; 95% CI: 1.18 to 4.76) and may be considered in refractory cases.[31]

Proton Pump Inhibitors

As uncontrolled gastroesophageal reflux may initiate or potentiate tendencies toward NVP, control of reflux has been associated with decreased severity of symptoms and increased quality of life. Aluminum or calcium antacids are first-line agents for symptomatic control. Products containing magnesium should not be used due to association with fetal respiratory distress, hypotonia, and nephrolithiasis. Therapies containing bicarbonates are associated with maternal/fetal alkalosis and fluid overload and are therefore not recommended. H2 blockers and proton pump inhibitors are considered safe for use during pregnancy.[32,33]

Corticosteroids

The role of steroids in the treatment of NVP is controversial and is typically reserved for only refractory NVP or HG. Although the exact dosage/regimen is unknown, a suggested regimen of methylprednisolone equivalent to 48 mg orally or intravenously in 3 divided doses per day for a 48- to 72-hour trial with discontinuation thereafter if ineffective has been proposed. If effective, the dose may be tapered over 1 to 2 weeks with continuation of the lowest effective dose for approximately 6 weeks. A prolonged course of steroids is not recommended due to potential adverse effects to the mother, including glucose intolerance.[34,35] An increased rate of cleft palate (up to 3.4-fold) and other major malformations after exposure during the first trimester has been established, prompting some to recommend its use in refractory cases only after 10 weeks gestation.[36-39]

COMPLEMENTARY/ALTERNATIVE

ACUPRESSURE/NEUROMODULATORS

Complementary/alternative approaches, such as acupressure, have been studied with equivocal results. According to Chinese medicine, pericardium 6 (P6), an acupoint located approximately 4.5 cm above the wrist on the inside of the forearm, is integral to relieving nausea and emesis. Through manual pressure or mechanical neurostimulators such as PrimaBella (Alaven Pharmaceutical LLC, Marietta, GA), an FDA-cleared neurostimulator with an indication for NVP, stimulation of the median nerve emits signals to the vomiting center in the brain and is thought to reset aberrant gastric pacing activity to improve nausea. Although the impact is not proven, some studies have shown up to a 50% response when compared to placebo, while others show no benefit over sham procedure.[40] Auricular acupressure and acupuncture have not been shown to reduce symptoms in recent trials.[41,42] Therefore, acupressure is considered an unproven, but safe and noninvasive intervention.[43]

GINGER

In addition to the use of preconception multivitamins as a preventative measure, ACOG also supports the use of ginger capsules as therapy for NVP. Ginger intake is associated with increased gastrointestinal motility and secretion of digestive fluids throughout the GI tract (saliva, gastric secretions, and bile). Additionally, it is thought to have an antiemetic effect similar to the $5\text{-}HT_3$ antagonist ondansetron and may play a role in inhibiting the growth of *H pylori*.[27] Typical therapeutic doses range from 1 to 2 g/day in divided doses, but optimal dosing and duration is unknown. Although there are no formal studies to assess potential adverse fetal outcomes, the effects of ginger on thromboxane synthetase and subsequent inhibition of platelet aggregation as well as inhibition of testosterone binding raise potential concerns. The effects on platelet aggregation pose a theoretical concern for increased risk of peripartum bleeding in both mother and fetus, particularly when other anticoagulants are prescribed or inherent bleeding tendencies are known; however, in doses of 1 g or less, no adverse events were reported.[44,45]

NUTRITIONAL CONSIDERATIONS

In cases of refractory NVP and HG, intravenous hydration to avoid or correct dehydration and electrolyte disturbances may be required. Infusion of thiamine is recommended to reduce the potential risk of Wernicke's encephalopathy. If caloric deficits are noted in association with concern for intrauterine growth retardation, implementation of nasogastric or nasojejunal feedings may be considered but are limited by aesthetics; durability of placement, especially in the setting of ongoing symptoms; and potential symptom provocation by tube feed infusion. There are limited reports of percutaneous gastrostomy and surgical jejunostomy tube placements for refractory symptoms, but these options should be considered for only the most severe cases.[46,47] In severe cases, parenteral nutrition may be required for the term of the pregnancy, but carries the risk of significant morbidity as a consequence of line infections as well as increased risk of fetal complications when compared with those receiving enteral supportive care. Rates of peripheral catheter complications are lower than those of central catheters, but are not insignificant (9% and 50%, respectively), with 25% risk of line sepsis.[48,49] Although there is no evidence to support any dietary recommendations in the treatment of NVP, folate supplementation should be instituted in cases of severe NVP and HG.

SUMMARY

NVP is a common condition affecting the majority of gravid women in early pregnancy. Although the pathophysiology is not well understood, multiple theories exist. As the condition is self-limited and mild in the majority of pregnancies, dietary and lifestyle changes may be effective in modifying symptoms, but pharmacologic therapies are helpful and safe in the majority of patients (Table 2-1). Unfortunately, treatment interventions for severe nausea and HG are limited and inconsistently effective, but should be used early in the presentation of the condition in an attempt to minimize the psychological and medical morbidity to both mother and fetus while potentially reducing the financial burden associated with NVP.[50]

Table 2-1

Pharmacologic Treatments of Nausea and Vomiting of Pregnancy

Medication	FDA Category*	Dose	Pregnancy Comment
Vitamin B$_6$ (pyridoxine)	A/C	10 to 25 mg PO q8hr	Safety is verified in low doses.
Pyridoxine-doxylamine	A/C	Pyridoxine 10 to 25 mg PO q8hr; doxylamine 25 mg PO at bedtime with 12.5 mg in the morning and afternoon PRN	Exact dose/interval of doxylamine may vary if compounded. Supplied OTC as Unisom SleepTabs or in delayed release formulation. SE: Sedation
Antihistamines			
Doxylamine (Unisom SleepTabs)	A	12.5 to 25 mg PO q8hr	SE: Sedation
Diphenhydramine (Benadryl)	B	25 to 50 mg PO q4 to 6 hr or 10 to 50 mg IV q4 to 6 hr	SE: Sedation
Meclizine (Bonine)	B	25 mg PO q4 to 6hr	SE: Sedation
Hydroxyzine (Atarax, Vistaril)	C	50 to 100 mg PO/PR q4 to 6hr	SE: Sedation
Dimenhydrinate (Dramamine)	B	50 to 100 mg PO/IV q4 to 6hr	SE: Sedation
Phenothiazines			
Promethazine (Phenergan)	C	25 mg PO/IM/PR q4 to 6 hr	SE: Sedation, extrapyramidal symptoms

(continued)

Table 2-1 *(continued)*

Pharmacologic Treatments of Nausea and Vomiting of Pregnancy

Medication	FDA Category*	Dose	Pregnancy Comment
Prochlorperazine (Compazine)	C	5 to 12.5 mg PO/IV/IM q6hr	Also available as rectal suppository. SE: Sedations, Extrapyramidal symptoms
Dopamine Antagonists			
Metoclopramide (Reglan)	B	10 mg PO/IV/ IM q6hr	Increased risk of tardive dyskinesia after more than 3 months of treatment. (Black-box warning)
Droperidol (Inapsine)	C	1.25 to 2.5 mg IM/IV	Torsades de pointes and cardiac arrhythmias— serial EKGs recommended. QT prolongation (Black-box warning).
Other			
Serotonin Antagonist Ondansetron (Zofran)	B	4 to 8 mg PO q6hr	SE: Constipation, diarrhea, dizziness, headache, drowsiness

(continued)

Table 2-1 *(continued)*

Pharmacologic Treatments of
Nausea and Vomiting of Pregnancy

Medication	FDA Category*	Dose	Pregnancy Comment
Glucocorticoid Methylprednisolone	C	16 mg PO q8hr x 3 days then taper over 1 to 2 weeks if initially effective.	Avoid prolonged use (>6 wks) to avoid maternal complications. SE: Slight increase in incidence of cleft lip/palate if used at less than 10 wks gestational age.
Ginger	C	125 to 250 mg PPO q6hr	SE: Reflux, heartburn

Adapted from Niebyl JR. Nausea and vomiting in pregnancy. *N Engl J Med.* 2011;363:1544-1550.

*See Appendix for discussion of FDA pregnancy categories.

REFERENCES

1. Lee N, Saha S. Nausea and vomiting of pregnancy. *Gastroenterol Clin North Am.* 2011;40:309-344.
2. Lacasse A, Rey E, Ferreira E, Morin C, Bérard A. Epidemiology of nausea and vomiting of pregnancy: prevalence, severity, determinants, and the importance of race/ethnicity. *BMC Pregnancy and Childbirth.* 2009;9:26-34.
3. Klebanoff M, Koslowe P, Kaslow R, Rhoads GG. Epidemiology of vomiting in early pregnancy. *Obstet Gynecol.* 1985;66:612-616.
4. Davis M. Nausea and vomiting of pregnancy: an evidence based review. *J Perinatal Neonatal Nursing.* 2004;18:312-328.
5. Mori M, Amino N, Tamaki K, Miyai K, Tanizawa O. Morning sickness and thyroid function in normal pregnancy. *Obstet Gynecol.* 1988;72:355-359.
6. Yoneyama Y, Suzuki S, Sawa R, et al. The T-helper 1/T-helper 2 balance in the peripheral blood of women with hyperemesis gravidarum. *Am J Obstet Gynecol.* 2002;187:1631-1635.
7. Goldberg D, Szilagyi A, Graves L. Hyperemesis gravidarum and *Helicobacter pylori* infection. *Obstet Gynecol.* 2007;110:695-703.

8. Tierson FD, Olsen CL, Hook EB. Nausea and vomiting of pregnancy and association with pregnancy outcome. *Am J Obstet Gynecol.* 1986;155: 1017-1023.

9. Weigel MM, Weigel RM. The association of reproductive history, demographic factors, and alcohol and tobacco consumption with the risk of developing nausea and vomiting in early pregnancy. *Am J Epidemiol.* 1988;127:562-570.

10. Flaxman SM, Sherman PW. Morning sickness: a mechanism for protecting mother and embryo. *Quarterly Rev Biol.* 2000;75:113-148.

11. Trogstad LI, Stoltenberg C, Magnus P, Skjaerven R, Irgens LM. Recurrence risk in hyperemesis gravidarum. *BJOG.* 2005;112(12):1641-1645.

12. Yoneyama Y, Suzuki S, Sawa R, Araki T. Plasma adenosine concentrations increase in women with hyperemesis gravidarum. *Clin Chim Acta.* 2004;342: 99-103.

13. Leylek OA, Toyaksi M, Erselcan T, Dokmetas S. Immunologic and biochemical factors in hyperemesis gravidarum with or without hyperthyroxinemia. *Gynecol Obstet Invest.* 1999;47:229-234.

14. Sanu O, Lamont RF. Hyperemesis gravidarum: pathogenesis and the use of antiemetic agents. *Expert Opin Pharmacother.* 2011;12(5):737-748.

15. Fell DB, Dodds L, Joseph KS, Allen VM, Butler B. Risk factors for hyperemesis gravidarum requiring hospital admission during pregnancy. *Obstet Gynecol.* 2006;107:277-284.

16. Jarvis S, Nelson-Piercy C. Management of nausea and vomiting in pregnancy. *BMJ.* 2011;17:342.

17. O'Mahony S. Endoscopy in pregnancy. *Best Pract Res Clin Gastroenterol.* 2007;21(5):893-899.

18. Niebyl JR. Nausea and vomiting in pregnancy. *N Engl J Med.* 2010;363: 1544-1550.

19. Jednak MA, Shadigian EM, Kim MS, et al. Protein meals reduce nausea and gastric slow wave dysrhythmic activity in the first trimester of pregnancy. *Am J Physiol.* 1999;277(4, pt 1):G855-G861.

20. Einarson A, Maltepe C, Boskovic R, Koren G. Treatment of nausea and vomiting in pregnancy: an updated algorithm. *Can Family Phys.* 2007;53(12): 2109-2111.

21. Arsenault MY, Lane CA. The management of nausea and vomiting of pregnancy. *J Obstet Gynaecol Can.* 2002;24(10):817-823.

22. Sahakian V, Rouse D, Sipes S, Rose N, Niebyl J. Vitamin B6 is effective therapy for nausea and vomiting of pregnancy: a randomized, double-blind placebo-controlled study. *Obstet Gynecol.* 1991;78(1):33-36.

23. Vutyavanich T, Wongtra-ngan S, Ruangsri R. Pyridoxine for nausea and vomiting of pregnancy: a randomized, double-blind, placebo-controlled trial. *Am J Obstet Gynecol.* 1995;173:881-884.

24. Tan PC, Yow CM, Omar SZ. A placebo-controlled trial of oral pyridoxine in hyperemesis gravidarum. *Gynecol Obstet Invest.* 2009;67:151-157.

25. McKeigue PM, Lamm SH, Linn S, Kutcher JS. Bendectin and birth defects: I. A meta-analysis of the epidemiologic studies. *Teratology.* 1994;50(1):27-37.

26. Badell ML, Ramin SM, Smtih JA. Treatment options for nausea and vomiting during pregnancy. *Pharmacotherapy.* 2006;26(9):1273-1287.

27. Matok I, Gorodischer R, Koren G, Sheiner E, Wiznitzer A, Levy A. The safety of metoclopramide use in the first trimester of pregnancy. *N Engl J Med.* 2009;360(24):2528-2535.

28. Rumeau-Rouquette C, Goujard J, Huel G. Possible teratogenic effect of phenothiazines in human beings. *Teratology.* 1977;15(1):57-64.

29. Tan PC, Khine PP, Vallikkannu N, Omar SZ. Promethazine compared with metoclopramide for hyperemesis gravidarum. *Obstet Gynecol.* 2002;115(5): 975-981.

30. Nageotte MP, Briggs GG, Towers CV, Asrat T. Droperidol and diphenhydramine in the management of hyperemesis gravidarum. *Am J Obstet Gynecol.* 1996;174(6):1801-1805.

31. Anderka M, Mitchell AA, Louik C, Werler MM, Hernandez-Diaz S, Rasmussen SA. National Birth Defects Prevention Study. Medications used to treat nausea and vomiting of pregnancy and the risk of selected birth defects. *Birth Defects Res A Clin Mol Teratol.* 2012;94(1):22-30.

32. Gill SK, O'Brien L, Koren G. The safety of histamine 2 (H2) blockers in pregnancy: a meta-analysis. *Dig Dis Sci.* 2009;54:1835-1838.

33. Gill SK, O'Brien LO, Einarson TR, Koren G. The safety of proton pump inhibitors (PPIs) in pregnancy: a meta-analysis. *Am J Gastroenterol.* 2009;104: 1541-1545.

34. Chan GCP, Wilson AM. Complications of the use of corticosteroids for the treatment of hyperemesis gravidarum. *Br J Obstet Gynaecol.* 1995;102(6): 507-508.

35. Safari HR, Fassett MJ, Souter IC, Alsulyman OM, Goodwin TM. The efficacy of methylprednisolone in the treatment of hyperemesis gravidarum: a randomized, double-blind, controlled study. *Am J Obstet Gynecol.* 1998;179(4):921-924.

36. Park-Wyllie L, Mazzotta P, Pastuszak A, et al. Birth defects after maternal exposure to corticosteroids: prospective cohort study and meta-analysis of epidemiological studies. *Teratology.* 2000;62(6):385-392.

37. Carmichael SL, Shaw GM. Maternal corticosteroid use and risk of selected congenital anomalies. *Am J Med Genet.* 1999;86(3):242-244.

38. Rodriguez-Pinilla E, Martinez-Frias ML. Corticosteroids during pregnancy and oral clefts: a case-control study. *Teratology.* 1998;58(1):2-5.

39. Ebrahimi N, Maltepe C, Einarson A. Optimal management of nausea and vomiting of pregnancy. *Int J Women's Health.* 2010;2:241-248.

40. Heazell A, Thorneycroft J, Walton V, Etherington I. Acupressure for the inpatient treatment of nausea and vomiting in early pregnancy: a randomized control trial. *Am J Obstet Gynecol.* 2006;194(3):815-820.

41. Puangsricharern A, Mahasukhon S. Effectiveness of auricular acupressure in the treatment of nausea and vomiting in early pregnancy. *J Med Assoc Thai.* 2008;91:1633-1638.

42. Smith C, Crowther C, Beilby J. Acupuncture to treat nausea and vomiting in early pregnancy: a randomized controlled trial. *Birth.* 2002;29(1):1-9.

43. Ernst E, Lee MS, Choi TY. Acupuncture in obstetrics and gynecology: an overview of systematic reviews. *Am J Chin Med.* 2011;39(3):423-431.

44 White B. Ginger: an overview. *Am Family Physician.* 2007;75:46-52.

45. Matthews A, Dowsell T, Haas DM, Doyle M, O'Mathúna DP. Interventions for nausea and vomiting in early pregnancy. *Cochrane Database of Systematic Reviews.* 2010;9:Art. No.: CD007575.

46. Barclay BA. Experience with enteral nutrition in the treatment of hyperemesis gravidarum. *Nutr Clin Prac.* 1990;5:153-155.
47. Saha S, Loranger D, Pricolo V, Degli-Esposti S. Feeding jejunostomy for the treatment of severe hyperemesis gravidarum: a case series. *J Parenteral Enteral Nutr.* 2009;33:529-534.
48. Folk JJ, Leslie-Brown HR, Nosovitch JT, Silverman RK, Aubry RH. Hyperemsis gravidarum: outcomes and complications with and without total parenteral nutrition. *J Reprod Med.* 2004;49:497-502.
49. Russo-Stieglitz KE, Levine AB, Wagner BA, Armenti VT. Pregnancy outcomes in patients requiring parenteral nutrition. *J Maternal Fetal Med.* 1999;8:164-167.
50. Tan PC, Vani S, Lim BK, Omar SZ. Anxiety and depression in hyperemesis gravidarum: prevalence, risk factors and correlation with clinical severity. *Eur J Obstet Gynecol Reprod Biol.* 2010;149:153-158.

3

Gastric Bypass and Pregnancy

D. Wayne Overby, MD

One-third of Americans older than 20 years are obese. Obesity is defined as having a Body Mass Index (BMI, calculated as weight in kilograms divided by height in square meters) greater than 30 kg/m^2. The prevalence of obesity is even higher among women, at 35.5%.[1] Weight loss surgery is the most effective treatment for morbid obesity (BMI >40 or >35 with an obesity-related comorbidity) and for obesity-related health problems.[2-4] The number of weight loss procedures performed per year in the United States has grown significantly over the past 20 years. In 1990, about 12,000 bariatric procedures were performed with a rate of 2.7 per 100,000 adults; the number of procedures peaked at about 135,000, 63.9 per 100,000, in 2004; and finally plateaued at 124,000, 54.2 per 100,000, in 2008.[5] Roux-en-Y gastric bypass (RYGB) accounted for 99% of operations in 2003, but declined to 69% of operations in 2008, when about 30% of the procedures performed were laparoscopic adjustable gastric banding (LAGB)[1]; recent data suggest that LAGB has overtaken RYGB as the most commonly performed procedure, and laparoscopic sleeve gastrectomy is the third most common procedure.[6] The majority of bariatric surgery, about 83%, is done in women, and women of

Isaacs KL, Long MD.
GI and Liver Disease During Pregnancy:
A Practical Approach (pp. 31-38).
© 2013 Taylor & Francis Group

reproductive age (18 to 45 years) account for about half of all weight loss procedures.[5,7] Obesity increases the risk of infertility and sub-fertility (increased time-to-pregnancy).[8,9] Weight loss after bariatric surgery results in an increase in fertility,[10] and female patients in this age group should be made aware of this and counseled regarding contraception. Providers should also be aware of the increased likeli-hood of encountering pregnant patients after gastric bypass.

KEY POINTS
• Obesity increases risk of infertility and subfertility.
• Weight loss after bypass increases fertility.

PATHOPHYSIOLOGY

Gastric bypass for weight loss has two main components: 1) the reduction of stomach capacity by creating a small (usually <30 mL) gastric pouch that is divided away from the rest of the stomach and 2) food bypassing the duodenum and first portion of the jejunum. Food instead empties from the gastric pouch and is carried downstream by a limb of jejunum, which makes up one side of the "Y"-shaped reconstruction (the Roux or alimentary limb). Undigested food then empties into the mid-jejunum, where it mixes with bile and pancreatic secretions from the other side of the "Y" (the biliopancreatic limb). Joining the 2 limbs at the jejuno-jejunostomy, the crotch of the "Y," creates a distal common channel for absorption. The classic explanation for weight loss after gastric bypass emphasizes the importance of the restriction of food intake by the small gastric pouch, in combination with decreased absorp-tion of calories as a result of bypassing part of the small bowel, but there is growing evidence to suggest more complex mechanisms involving changes in gut hormones and metabolism.[11] The surgical alteration of normal anatomy is not easily reversed and should be considered permanent.

Most experts recommend avoiding pregnancy for at least 1 year and as many as 2 years after gastric bypass, the period during which the most rapid weight loss occurs.[12,13] This delay is recommended both to protect the developing fetus from possible complications related to immediate postgastric bypass physiologic milieu and to optimize the mother's weight loss. Data regarding pregnancy soon after gastric bypass are limited, but if pregnancy does occur during this period, it may not cause increased risks to mother and fetus.[13-15]

KEY POINT
• Avoid pregnancy for 1 to 2 years after gastric bypass to allow weight to stabilize.

While there have been relatively few studies of pregnancy after gastric bypass, and while most studies are small and often have conflicting results, pregnancy after gastric bypass seems to pose little additional risk to the mother, and the weight lost after gastric bypass seems to make the rates of gestational diabetes, hypertensive complications, and delivery-related complications similar to those of controls.[13-16] When pregnancies occurring in the same patient before and after RYGB are compared, there is less weight gained by patients post-RYGB, and the weight gained with pregnancy may be lost more quickly.[17]

KEY POINTS
• There is less weight gain with pregnancy after gastric bypass.
• Weight gain with pregnancy is lost more quickly postbypass.

COMPLICATIONS IN PREGNANT GASTRIC BYPASS PATIENTS

Surgical complications resulting from gastric bypass in pregnant patients, such as small-bowel obstruction related to internal hernia, and gastrojejunostomy ulcers or strictures, have been reported. These complications carry the risk of maternal death and fetal loss and can require emergent surgical treatment, including the need for laparoscopic or open abdominal exploration and unplanned cesarean section (C-section). Pregnant patients may experience delays in diagnosis and treatment when symptoms are vague or confounded by pregnancy, and providers are reluctant to order studies that rely on ionizing radiation. As suggested by one author, reports of fetal and maternal death as a result of complications due to gastric bypass "underscore the need for prompt diagnosis and management for women treated by bypass surgery presenting with abdominal pain during pregnancy; if required, no examination is contraindicated during pregnancy, including computed tomography with iodine injection."[16,18]

KEY POINT

- Promptly evaluate abdominal pain in patients with gastric bypass.

NUTRITIONAL ISSUES IN GASTRIC BYPASS PATIENTS

While clinically evident malnutrition after RYGB is relatively rare, micronutrient deficiencies are a valid concern. The most common nutritional abnormalities after gastric bypass are deficiencies of protein; iron; calcium; and vitamins D, B_{12}, and folate. Several studies have reported nutrition-related problems in pregnant patients after gastric bypass; some found low rates of anemia, up to 11%, and some reported neural tube defects in mothers not adherent to supplements. However, other studies have failed to find increased rates of anemia or neural tube defects in mothers having children after gastric bypass.[7,15,16,18,19]

KEY POINTS

- Check albumin; iron; calcium; and vitamins D, B_{12}, and folate.
- Ensure adequate folate supplementation to prevent neural tube defects.

There is no difference in rates of premature delivery following gastric bypass. The results regarding rates of low birth weight are mixed, with some studies suggesting lower birth weight in children born to mothers who have had gastric bypass; rates of macrosomia are similar to those of controls.[7,13,16,18,19] Some studies report a higher rate of C-section in mothers after gastric bypass, but this may reflect repeat C-sections in patients who have had previous C-sections.[18]

KEY POINT
• Delivery method is based on obstetric indications.

MANAGEMENT

Because there are so few data, care during pregnancy of mothers who have undergone gastric bypass requires a common-sense approach, with principles based both on standard prenatal care and on the care of nonpregnant patients who have had gastric bypass. It is important to note that the usual testing for gestational diabetes in patients after gastric bypass can be complicated by dumping syndrome, which can cause significant intolerance to oral intake of foods or drinks high in simple sugars; serial comparisons of fasting and postprandial blood glucose levels or glycosylated hemoglobin levels can be substituted instead. Baseline laboratory studies should be obtained and repeated each trimester, including complete blood count (CBC), electrolytes, glucose, iron studies, folate levels, and levels of vitamins D and B_{12}, with deficiencies replaced as needed. Regular supplementation should include a prenatal vitamin (PNV), calcium 1200 mg/day, with vitamin D 400 to 800 U/day, the usual daily PNV dose of folate of 400 µg, 40 to 65 mg/day of elemental iron, and oral B_{12} 350 µg/day. Protein intake should be 60 to 70 g/day. Total caloric intake should be sufficient to allow recommended levels of weight gain.[20] The high-risk obstetrical specialist, bariatric surgeon, and nutritionist should be consulted as needed.

KEY POINTS
• Follow CBC; electrolyes; glucose; iron; folate; and vitamins D and B_{12} each trimester.
• Use regular oral supplementation:
∞ PNV—standard dosing one per day
∞ Calcium—1200 mg/day   *(continued)*

KEY POINTS *(continued)*
∞ Vitamin D—400 to 800 U/day
∞ Folate—400 µg/day
∞ Elemental iron—40 to 65 mg/day
∞ B_{12}—350 µg/day
• Protein intake should be 60 to 70 g/day

SUMMARY

While data regarding the implications of gastric bypass on pregnant patients continue to accrue, clinicians are obligated to care for them and make decisions, regardless of the current state of the art. That being said, available studies do suggest that patients and providers should expect a comparatively normal pregnancy and delivery without undue fetal risk, and, while not recommended, this seems to be true even if pregnancy occurs soon after surgery. The weight lost after gastric bypass decreases the risk of many complications associated with obesity in pregnancy, and it serves to improve most outcomes. Unavoidably, pregnant patients who have had weight loss surgery will be increasingly common. A sensible approach to prenatal care, nutrition, and delivery, along with a high index of suspicion in patients with symptoms indicative of possible complications, can lead to good results for mother and fetus.

REFERENCES

1. Flegal KM, Carroll MD, Ogden CL, Curtin LR. Prevalence and trends in obesity among US adults, 1999-2008. *JAMA.* 2010;303(3):235-241.
2. Maggard MA, Shugarman LR, Suttorp M, et al. Meta-analysis: surgical treatment of obesity. *Ann Intern Med.* 2005;142(7):547-559.
3. Colquitt JL, Picot J, Loveman E, Clegg AJ. Surgery for obesity. *Cochrane Database Syst Rev.* 2009;15(2):CD003641.
4. Buchwald H, Avidor Y, Braunwald E, et al. Bariatric surgery: a systematic review and meta-analysis. *JAMA.* 2004;292(14):1724-1737.
5. Nguyen NT, Masoomi H, Magno CP, Nguyen XM, Laugenour K, Lane J. Trends in use of bariatric surgery, 2003-2008. *J Am Coll Surg.* 2011;213(2): 261-266.
6. Hutter MM, Schirmer BD, Jones DB, et al. First report from the American College of Surgeons Bariatric Surgery Center Network: laparoscopic sleeve gastrectomy has morbidity and effectiveness positioned between the band and the bypass. *Ann Surg.* 2011;254(3):410-420, discussion 20-22.

7. Maggard MA, Yermilov I, Li Z, et al. Pregnancy and fertility following bariatric surgery: a systematic review. *JAMA*. 2008;300(19):2286-2296.

8. Gesink Law DC, Maclehose RF, Longnecker MP. Obesity and time to pregnancy. *Hum Reprod*. 2007;22(2):414-420.

9. Nohr EA, Vaeth M, Rasmussen S, Ramlau-Hansen CH, Olsen J. Waiting time to pregnancy according to maternal birthweight and prepregnancy BMI. *Hum Reprod*. 2009;24(1):226-232.

10. Nelson SM, Fleming R. Obesity and reproduction: impact and interventions. *Curr Opin Obstet Gynecol*. 2007;19(4):384-389.

11. Ochner CN, Gibson C, Shanik M, Goel V, Geliebter A. Changes in neurohormonal gut peptides following bariatric surgery. *Int J Obes (Lond)*. 2011;35(2):153-166.

12. American College of Obstetricians and Gynecologists. ACOG Committee Opinion number 315, September 2005. Obesity in pregnancy. *Obstet Gynecol*. 2005;106(3):671-675.

13. Patel JA, Patel NA, Thomas RL, Nelms JK, Colella JJ. Pregnancy outcomes after laparoscopic Roux-en-Y gastric bypass. *Surg Obes Relat Dis*. 2008;4(1): 39-45.

14. Dao T, Kuhn J, Ehmer D, Fisher T, McCarty T. Pregnancy outcomes after gastric-bypass surgery. *Am J Surg*. 2006;192(6):762-766.

15. Wax JR, Cartin A, Wolff R, Lepich S, Pinette MG, Blackstone J. Pregnancy following gastric bypass surgery for morbid obesity: maternal and neonatal outcomes. *Obes Surg*. 2008;18(5):540-544.

16. Sheiner E, Balaban E, Dreiher J, Levi I, Levy A. Pregnancy outcome in patients following different types of bariatric surgeries. *Obes Surg*. 2009;19(9):1286-1292.

17. Wittgrove AC, Jester L, Wittgrove P, Clark GW. Pregnancy following gastric bypass for morbid obesity. *Obes Surg*. 1998;8(4):461-464; discussion 465-466.

18. Santulli P, Mandelbrot L, Facchiano E, et al. Obstetrical and neonatal outcomes of pregnancies following gastric bypass surgery: a retrospective cohort study in a French referral centre. *Obes Surg*. 2010;20(11):1501-1508.

19. Sapre N, Munting K, Pandita A, Stubbs R. Pregnancy following gastric bypass surgery: what is the expected course and outcome? *N Z Med J*. 2009;122(1306):33-42.

20. Kominiarek MA. Pregnancy after bariatric surgery. *Obstet Gynecol Clin North Am*. 2010;37(2):305-320.

4

Abdominal Pain in Pregnancy

Differential Diagnosis and Initial Work-Up of Abdominal Pain

Millie D. Long, MD, MPH

While many of the principles of diagnosing and treating a woman with abdominal pain do not change due to pregnancy, the prevalence of several important causes of abdominal pain can be affected by the pregnancy itself. While the differential diagnosis of abdominal pain can be similar regardless of pregnancy, the risk/benefit ratio of certain diagnostic tests can change. Therefore, the work-up of abdominal pain in a pregnant woman includes a delicate balance. However, concern about the possible fetal effects of radiation should not prevent medically indicated diagnostic testing during pregnancy. In general, the well-being of the mother takes precedence, as proper treatment of the mother will benefit the fetus.

Isaacs KL, Long MD.
*GI and Liver Disease During Pregnancy:
A Practical Approach (pp. 39-60).*
© 2013 Taylor & Francis Group

Physiologic Changes Affecting the Gastrointestinal Tract During Pregnancy

There are many physiologic changes during pregnancy, including an increase of 35% to 50% of blood volume, cardiac output, and heart rate. Many of the physiologic changes of pregnancy can directly affect the gastrointestinal tract. For example, lower esophageal sphincter (LES) tone is reduced during pregnancy, thereby increasing reflux. Reduced progesterone levels and other changes in sex hormones are thought to affect not only LES tone, but also bowel motility[1,2] and gallbladder emptying.[3] Pregnancy itself predisposes to gallstone formation, and biliary tract diseases can therefore be common during pregnancy. Also, venous thrombosis risk is increased during pregnancy related to venous stasis, endothelial injury, and the underlying hypercoagulable state. Acute vascular events, such as a pulmonary thrombotic embolism, can present as upper abdominal pain. Infectious risks are increased with pregnancy, and infections of the genitourinary or pulmonary tract can manifest as abdominal pain. Other disorders specific to pregnancy, such as morning sickness, can be confused with acute gastrointestinal disorders. An additional factor influencing the work-up of abdominal pain in pregnancy is that the gravid uterus can compress the viscera and abdominal wall.[4] This compression can alter the sensation and localization of pain. Therefore, the locations of pain classically seen in the nonpregnant patient may not hold in a pregnant patient.

Key Questions

There are key questions to ask in the evaluation of a pregnant woman with abdominal pain (Table 4-1). These questions should include characteristics of the pregnancy (such as fetal movement [if applicable] and vaginal bleeding), characteristics of the abdominal pain (such as onset, location, intensity, character, and exacerbating factors), and other associated symptoms. In particular, the presence of fever should be assessed. Other symptoms that can help to differentiate the cause of abdominal pain include whether the patient has nausea/vomiting, rectal bleeding, weight loss, or a change in bowel habits. These questions, combined with physical examination and appropriate diagnostic testing, can help to differentiate the cause of the abdominal pain.

Table 4-1

Key Questions

• Characteristics of the pregnancy
  ∞ Fetal movement (if applicable)
  ∞ Vaginal bleeding
• Characteristics of the pain
  ∞ Location
  ∞ Onset
  ∞ Severity
  ∞ Character
  ∞ Anything that exacerbates or improves the pain
  ∞ Any history of similar pain prior to pregnancy
• Presence of fever
• Nausea and vomiting
• Weight loss
• Rectal bleeding/blood in stool
• Changes in bowel habits
  ∞ Diarrhea
  ∞ Constipation

The differential diagnosis and initial work-up of abdominal pain in a pregnant woman can be divided into pregnancy-related and non–pregnancy-related causes. This chapter will focus on the non–pregnancy-related causes of abdominal pain. The prevalence, classic symptoms, and appropriate diagnostic work-up will be discussed for each potential etiology of non–pregnancy-related abdominal pain.

PREGNANCY-RELATED CAUSES OF ABDOMINAL PAIN

There are several normal physiologic components of pregnancy that can be associated with abdominal pain. Some of these normal components of pregnancy include pain associated with the enlarging uterus, fetal movement triggering pain, round ligament pain, and contractions.

KEY POINTS

- Normal pregnancy-related etiologies of abdominal pain include the following:
  - ∞ Enlarging uterus
  - ∞ Fetal movement
  - ∞ Round ligament pain
  - ∞ Contractions

Other pregnancy-related causes of pain are not normal and require immediate recognition and early therapy. These include ectopic pregnancy, uterine rupture, placental abruption, and miscarriage. Many of these entities present with pelvic or back pain, vaginal bleeding, uterine contractions, nonreassuring fetal tracing, and even maternal shock. Ectopic pregnancy is the most common obstetric cause of death in pregnancy.[4,5] Appropriate diagnostic evaluations can include laboratory assessments, such as CBC, ultrasonic evaluation, and fetal monitoring. Immediate therapy is indicated in these conditions.

KEY POINTS

- Pregnancy-related etiologies of abdominal pain requiring urgent evaluation include the following:
  - ∞ Ectopic pregnancy
  - ∞ Uterine rupture
  - ∞ Placental abruption
  - ∞ Miscarriage

Pregnancy-specific disorders of the liver can also present with right upper quadrant pain. These include hemolysis, elevated liver enzymes, low platelet syndrome (HELLP) and acute fatty liver of pregnancy (see Chapter 12). A pregnant woman with right upper quadrant pain should have an evaluation for pre-eclampsia with vital sign assessment and urinalysis. Additional investigations can include laboratory assessments of liver function tests (AST/ALT/ T Bili/Alk Phos), CBC, glucose, coagulation factors (PT/INR), and abdominal ultrasound.

KEY POINTS

- Pregnancy-related disoders of the liver include the following:
  - ∞ HELLP syndrome
  - ∞ Acute fatty liver of pregnancy

NON–PREGNANCY-RELATED CAUSES OF ABDOMINAL PAIN

Abdominal pain during pregnancy can arise from involvement of several different organ systems. Often, this arises from the gastrointestinal or hepatobiliary systems, but other causes can be gynecologic, genitourinary, vascular, or infectious. Establishing a complete differential diagnosis is necessary from the outset.

GASTROINTESTINAL

Gastrointestinal causes of abdominal pain are not necessarily more common during pregnancy but can be more difficult to diagnose and treat.

APPENDICITIS

Appendicitis is the most common indication for nonobstetric surgery during pregnancy. The incidence of appendicitis is 1 in 1500 pregnancies,[4,6] with a slight predilection for the second trimester. Diagnosing appendicitis during pregnancy can be difficult due to displacement upward of the appendix during pregnancy, limited physical examination due to the gravid uterus, and relatively imprecise laboratory evaluations. The patient's symptoms can be imprecise, including nausea, vomiting, and nonlocalizing abdominal pain. Peritoneal signs are less frequent, as the gravid uterus can lift the anterior abdominal wall away from the appendix. Fever is less common (~25%) among pregnant women with appendicitis.[7] However, the most common presenting symptom remains right lower quadrant abdominal pain.[8] Ultrasound can be used to visualize whether there is dilation or wall thickening of the appendix; however, this form of imaging is not ideal, particularly in a pregnant patient. Even in the nonpregnant adult population, the sensitivity ranges from 50% to 100%, specificity from 33% to 92%.[4] Therefore, a negative ultrasound does not necessarily correlate with lack of appendicitis. MRI is, therefore, often used if there is any question of the diagnosis after ultrasound is performed.[4] Diagnostic laparoscopy can also be used and has reduced the rate of false-positive appendectomy.[7] It is important to diagnose appendicitis prior to perforation, as perforation is associated with markedly increased risk of fetal loss and maternal mortality.

KEY POINTS

- Appendicitis occurs in 1 in 1500 pregnancies.
- Symptoms are imprecise and often include nausea, vomiting, and abdominal pain.
- Fever is less common among pregnant women with appendicitis.
- Initial work-up can include ultrasound, MRI, and diagnostic laparoscopy.

BOWEL OBSTRUCTION

Intestinal obstruction can also occur in pregnancy. The symptoms are relatively nonspecific, including nausea, vomiting, and abdominal pain. The diagnosis can be difficult, as the physical exam findings can be limited in the setting of a gravid uterus. The etiology of a bowel obstruction can be related to adhesions from prior surgeries, volvulus, intussusception, malignancy, inflammatory bowel disease, or hernias. Pregnant patients most often present with bowel obstruction in the third trimester. This may be related to the mass effect of the enlarging uterus causing displacement of the bowel. Ultrasound can find dilated loops of bowel with fluid levels and aperistalsis; however, ultrasound cannot usually determine whether there is a transition point.[4] Cross-sectional imaging via MRI can further characterize the cause of a bowel obstruction. If MRI cannot be performed, computed tomography (CT) may be performed in cases where there is suspicion for bowel obstruction, as delayed diagnosis and treatment of a potential bowel obstruction may pose a greater risk to the fetus than the radiation exposure from the CT.[4]

KEY POINTS

- Bowel obstruction is most common in the third trimester.
- Symptoms can include nausea, vomiting, and abdominal pain.
- Initial work-up can include ultrasound and MRI.

INFLAMMATORY BOWEL DISEASE

Inflammatory bowel disease (IBD) has a peak age of onset during the reproductive years. Therefore, a new diagnosis of IBD can occur during pregnancy with new onset of abdominal pain, rectal bleeding, diarrhea, and fever. Patients with underlying IBD can have flares of disease during pregnancy, which can also be associated with abdominal pain (see Chapter 7). Infectious etiologies also need to be ruled out in a patient presenting with these symptoms during pregnancy, regardless of whether there was a prior diagnosis of IBD. Other laboratory values, such as C-reactive protein and erythrocyte sedimentation rate, can be elevated during pregnancy and may not correlate with active inflammation. Ultrasound can demonstrate a thick-walled segment of bowel associated with active inflammation. MRI can also distinguish thick-walled bowel with stenosis and/or dilation. Distal endoscopic evaluations, such as flexible sigmoidoscopy, can be useful in order to obtain tissue diagnoses. Sigmoidoscopy procedures have been shown to be safe when indicated, particularly during the second trimester of pregnancy (see Chapter 8).[9] Recent data show that colonoscopy can be used during pregnancy in the second trimester when there is a strong indication, without worsened maternal or fetal outcomes.[10] In general, colonoscopy should be deferred if possible.

KEY POINTS
• Peak age of onset of IBD is during reproductive years, and initial symptoms can occur during pregnancy.
• Symptoms can include diarrhea, rectal bleeding, and abdominal pain.
• Infection should be ruled out with stool studies.
• Work-up can include abdominal ultrasound and flexible sigmoidoscopy (second trimester).

DIVERTICULITIS

Diverticulitis can occur among pregnant women. The symptoms typically consist of left lower quadrant pain, alteration in bowel habits, nausea, and fever. While white blood cell count can be elevated, this is not always the case. Complicated diverticulitis can occur, which is related to abscess, fistula, obstruction, or perforation. There are also case reports of diverticulitis arising from Meckel's diverticula in pregnant patients.[11,12] In the nonpregnant woman, the diagnostic test of choice is abdomen and pelvis CT scan. Endoscopic evaluation of the colon is deferred until after resolution of the diverticulitis, typically about 6 weeks after the episode. In the pregnant woman, initial work-up can include CBC, liver function tests, and abdominal ultrasound.

KEY POINTS
• Symptoms of diverticulitis can include left lower quadrant abdominal pain, nausea, and fever.
• Initial work-up can include CBC, liver function tests, and ultrasound.
• Endoscopic evaluation can be deferred until after delivery.

PEPTIC ULCER DISEASE

Peptic ulcer disease occurs less commonly in pregnancy, with less severe symptoms, and has fewer complications.[13] This may be partially related to recommendations for avoidance of nonsteroidal anti-inflammatory drugs (NSAIDs) during pregnancy. Symptoms of peptic ulcer disease include epigastric abdominal pain, burning, and nausea. Often, the diagnosis can be made based on response to therapy, as symptoms improve with antacid therapy. In cases of severe symptoms that are refractory to therapy, in the setting of gastrointestinal hemorrhage, and in suspected gastric outlet obstruction, upper endoscopy can be used in the pregnant patient (see Chapter 8). A severe complication of ulcer disease is perforation. Symptoms of perforation include severe diffuse abdominal pain, fever, and tachycardia peritoneal signs on exam. Suspicion of a perforation requires urgent surgical evaluation.

KEY POINTS
• Peptic ulcer disease is less common in pregnancy. • Symptoms include epigastric abdominal pain and burning. • Diagnosis is made by response to antacid therapy. • There is a role for endoscopy only in refractory cases or when there is bleeding.

GASTROESOPHAGEAL REFLUX DISEASE

Symptomatic gastroesophageal reflux disease (GERD) is common in pregnancy, with 40% to 80% of women experiencing symptoms of classic reflux.[14,15] This is related to reduced lower esophageal sphincter (LES) tone, likely associated with elevated levels of progesterone. Compromise of the weakened LES is also related to increased intra-abdominal pressure from the enlarging uterus. Symptoms can include a burning epigastric sensation that is worse after meals, regurgitation, and an acid brash taste. The onset is usually during the first or second trimester, and symptoms often continue throughout the pregnancy, with resolution after delivery.[7,13] Diagnosis is often made with response to lifestyle and dietary changes, antacids, H2 blockers, or proton pump inhibitors (see Chapter 1).

KEY POINTS
• GERD is common (~40% to 80% of all pregnant women). • Burning epigastric pain is worse after meals. • Diagnosis is made via response to antacid and lifestyle/dietary changes.

IRRITABLE BOWEL SYNDROME

Irritable bowel syndrome (IBS) is common in women of childbearing age,[16,17] although there are no large studies following the course of IBS through pregnancy. Diagnosis is made via history and physical examination, with a classic presentation. Patients often complain of chronic abdominal pain of variable intensity, which is associated with periods of acute exacerbation. The character, location, and severity of the pain vary significantly. Factors such as stress can exacerbate the pain. One classic feature of IBS is that the pain is often relieved with defecation. The abdominal pain is also often associated with changes in bowel habits, including diarrhea, constipation, or alternation of both diarrhea and constipation, often with a sensation of incomplete evacuation.[17] The Rome III criteria for diagnosis of IBS can aid in diagnosis.[18] Patients can also complain of nausea, increased bloating, and gas production. The diagnosis of IBS should be made in a classic presentation, with a lack of "red flag" symptoms. Symptoms of weight loss, bleeding, fever, and nocturnal awakening with pain and/or diarrhea warrant further investigation (see Chapter 6).

KEY POINTS
• IBS is intermittent abdominal pain relieved by defecation. • Patients with IBS have altered bowel habits. • There is a change in appearance of the stool. • There are no red flag symptoms.

HEPATOBILIARY

ACUTE CHOLECYSTITIS

Pregnancy predisposes to gallstone formation, and gallstones occur in approximately 7% of nulliparous women, but in 19% of women with two or more pregnancies.[7] The etiology is most likely related to biliary stasis, increased cholesterol synthesis, decreased gallbladder contraction, and prolonged intestinal transit.[4] Acute cholecystitis is rare in pregnancy (<1/8000),[7] but requires recognition and therapy. The classic symptoms of acute cholecystitis include right upper quadrant or epigastric pain, which can radiate to the back, and fever. Often, these symptoms are also associated with nausea and vomiting. The pain is usually preceded by ingestion of a fatty meal. Physical examination can demonstrate a positive Murphy's sign (pain with palpation of the gallbladder fossa beneath the liver edge, and associated inspiratory arrest). However, in the pregnant patient, this sign is less reliable. Laboratory evaluation with CBC, liver function tests, and ultrasound are the initial tests of choice.

KEY POINTS

- Acute cholecystitis is more common in multiparous women.
- Symptoms include right upper quadrant pain, fever, and nausea/vomiting.
- Symptoms are often preceded by a fatty meal.
- Initial work-up should include CBC, liver function tests, and abdominal ultrasound.

PANCREATITIS

Pancreatitis is rare in pregnancy (<1/8000) and is most often caused by gallstones. Pregnancy predisposes to gallstones for the reasons above. Additionally, higher levels of maternal estrogen are present in the third trimester, which can thereby increase triglyceride formation, resulting in a rare cause of pancreatitis. The symptoms of pancreatitis often include acute-onset upper abdominal pain, either in the right upper quadrant or epigastric region with radiation to the back. This is often accompanied by nausea, vomiting, and fever. Initial work-up includes CBC, liver function tests, and pancreatic enzymes (amylase/lipase). Amylase is less specific in pregnancy, and elevations are common related to pregnancy itself. Imaging of choice in the nonpregnant patient is contrast-enhanced CT. In the pregnant patient, imaging via ultrasound can be performed. Ultrasound can image the gallbladder and biliary tree; however, it is less useful in evaluating the pancreas. There can be overlying bowel gas obstructing the view. If ultrasound is normal or unequivocal, MRI/ magnetic resonance cholangiopancreatography (MRCP) is indicated to diagnose pancreatitis and search for potential causes, such as gallstones.[4]

> ### KEY POINTS
>
> - Patients can experience acute upper abdominal pain radiating to the back.
> - Symptoms include nausea, vomiting, and fever.
> - Initial work-up includes CBC, liver function tests, pancreatic enzymes, and ultrasound imaging of the biliary tree.

HEPATIC ADENOMA

Hepatic adenomas are benign tumors of the liver predominantly seen in young women. Abdominal pain in the right upper quadrant or epigastric region can arise with increasing size of the adenoma, bleeding into the tumor, or necrosis. Hepatic adenomas are associated with estrogen use and are influenced by increased steroid hormones during pregnancy. The size of the adenoma is a risk factor for rupture, which, in the pregnant patient, is associated with high maternal and fetal mortality. Symptoms of rupture can include sudden severe onset of pain associated with hypotension, which requires urgent therapy. Ultrasound is the initial test of choice and can characterize the size of the adenoma.

> ### KEY POINTS
>
> - Patients experience right upper quadrant abdominal pain.
> - Sudden severe pain with hypotension can be a sign of rupture.
> - Ultrasound is the diagnostic test of choice.

GENITOURINARY

NEPHROLITHIASIS

Kidney stones during pregnancy are rare, with an incidence of 1/1500 to 1/3000 pregnancies, usually presenting in the second or third trimester in a multiparous woman.[19] Pregnancy is associated with a mild increase in urinary calcium excretion, which may contribute to stone formation. Symptoms include flank pain with radiation to the groin or lower abdomen and hematuria. In the nonpregnant patient, a CT is often used for diagnosis. Testing of choice in the pregnant patient includes abdominal ultrasound followed by transvaginal ultrasound if needed. These tests are less sensitive than CT but are not associated with radiation exposure. Symptomatic improvement with intravenous hydration and positioning (affected side up, lying on the side) can also aid in the diagnosis of kidney stones.

KEY POINTS

- Nephrolithiasis is relatively rare during pregnancy.
- Symptoms include flank pain with radiation to the groin.
- Initial work-up can include urinalysis and abdominal ultrasound.

VASCULAR

PULMONARY VENOUS THROMBOEMBOLISM

Pregnancy is a state in which all three known risks for venous thrombosis coexist: venous stasis, endothelial injury, and a hypercoagulable state. Therefore, pregnancy itself is a risk factor for pulmonary venous thromboembolism (PE), occurring in 1 in 500 to 2000 pregnancies.[20,21] The risk for a venous thrombotic event is increased 5-fold in pregnancy and more than 60-fold in the postpartum period.[22] Deep venous thrombosis (DVT) is more common than actual PE. Interestingly, this is most common in the left leg due to compression of the left iliac vein by the right iliac artery and compression of the inferior vena cava by the gravid uterus. When PE does occur during pregnancy, it is equally distributed amongst the trimesters. Presenting symptoms of PE can include chest pain, abdominal pain, and shortness of breath. Both DVT and PE can be difficult to diagnose, as there is lower extremity swelling associated with pregnancy and dyspnea can occur with normal pregnancies. Laboratory assessments, including d-dimer, can be elevated in normal pregnancies. Initial assessments in a pregnant patient who is suspected of having a PE and/or DVT include Doppler ultrasound of the lower extremities and assessment of the clinical scenario/pretest probability of PE in order to determine whether a ventilation-perfusion scan or a specialized protocol CT should be performed.

KEY POINTS
• The risk of pulmonary embolism is increased 5-fold with pregnancy. • Symptoms include chest pain, abdominal pain, and shortness of breath. • Initial work-up includes Doppler ultrasound of the lower extremities.

SPLENIC ARTERY ANEURYSM

Splenic artery aneurysms are usually asymptomatic but can present with epigastric or left upper quadrant pain. Pregnancy is a risk factor for rupture of an aneurysm. This is thought to be related to hormonal changes that may alter elastic properties of the arterial wall.[4] Rupture can be catastrophic, associated with maternal and fetal mortality. Most often, these aneurysms are found incidentally. If an aneurysm is found incidentally in a woman of childbearing age, surgical intervention is recommended prior to pregnancy. Diagnostic imaging can detect these aneurysms, including ultrasound, CT, or MRI. In the pregnant patient, ultrasound is the initial test of choice.

KEY POINTS
• Splenic artery aneurysm is rare, often found incidentally. • Symptoms include left upper quadrant pain. • There is a risk of rupture during pregnancy. • Initial work-up includes abdominal ultrasound.

GYNECOLOGIC

ADNEXAL MASS

Adnexal mass occurs in only approximately 2% of all pregnancies and is usually not associated with pain.[23] If this becomes complicated by torsion, hemorrhage, or rupture, this can cause pain particularly in the right or left lower quadrant. Only 1% to 8% of those adnexal masses found during pregnancy are malignant.[4,24] Ultrasound is the initial imaging test of choice and can be followed by MRI if further characterization of a complex mass would change management during pregnancy.

KEY POINTS
• Adnexal mass occurs in 2% of all pregnancies.
• It is not painful unless complicated (torsion, rupture, etc).
• Symptoms can include right or left lower quadrant pain.
• Initial test of choice is abdominal ultrasound.

OVARIAN TORSION

Ovarian torsion complicates 1 in 800 pregnancies.[4] This can be associated with an adnexal mass or can simply occur in a normal ovary, typically on the right side.[24] This generally occurs between 6 and 14 weeks of gestation when uterine enlargement is most rapid, although it can occur at any point during pregnancy. The symptoms consist of lower quadrant abdominal pain, nausea, vomiting, low-grade fever, and leukocytosis. Laboratory assessment with CBC and imaging via ultrasound are the initial tests of choice.

KEY POINTS
• Ovarian torsion can be associated with adnexal mass.
• Symptoms can include lower quadrant abdominal pain, nausea, vomiting, and fever.
• Work-up includes laboratory assessment and abdominal ultrasound.

LEIOMYOMAS

Uterine leiomyomas can be common during pregnancy, and hospitalization for leiomyoma-related complications occurs in 1 in 500 pregnancies.[25] Abdominal pain and uterine contractions can result from rapid growth of leiomyomas and degeneration during pregnancy, particularly in the first trimester with rising estrogen levels. Patients can have pain as these leiomyomas increase in size (particularly >5 cm). The typical presentation consists of pain, but mild fever, nausea, and vomiting can also occur. Diagnosis is made via ultrasound. Ultrasound can confirm a degenerating leiomyoma as the source of pain, as often pain increases when the probe is placed directly over the leiomyoma.[25]

KEY POINTS
• Leiomyomas can be common.
• Symptoms include lower quadrant pain, fever, nausea, and vomiting.
• Diagnostic test of choice is ultrasound.

INFECTIOUS

PNEUMONIA

The incidence of pneumonia in pregnant women is similar to that of nonpregnant women, with a recent reported incidence of 1.2 to 2.7 per 1000 deliveries.[26] Changes during pregnancy that may be associated with increased susceptibility to infection include decreased lymphocyte proliferative response, decreased natural killer cell activity, changes in T cell populations, and reduced lymphocyte cytotoxic activity. Also, hormones present during pregnancy may inhibit cell-mediated immune function. The elevation of the diaphragm by the gravid uterus may also inhibit the mother's ability to clear secretions.[26] The classic presentation of pneumonia is fever, cough productive of sputum, and chest pain. However, in some women with lower lobe pneumonia, presentation can consist only of upper quadrant abdominal pain. Diagnosis of pneumonia in pregnancy is via physical examination, CBC, sputum culture, and chest x-ray. The small amount of radiation associated with a chest x-ray has not been associated with increased fetal malformations, and a diagnosis of pneumonia in a pregnant woman should not be missed. Pregnant women with pneumonia are more likely to develop pulmonary edema, as well as preterm labor and delivery.[27]

KEY POINTS

- Pregnant women may be more susceptible to infection.
- Symptoms include fever, cough, and chest or upper quadrant abdominal pain.
- Work-up includes examination, CBC, and chest x-ray.

URINARY TRACT INFECTION/ACUTE CYSTITIS/ PYELONEPHRITIS

Urinary tract infections are the most common infection during pregnancy. The incidence of asymptomatic bacteriuria is 2% to 10% during pregnancy. The incidence of acute cystitis is 1% to 4%.[28] Screening for asymptomatic bacteriuria is recommended during pregnancy, as treatment has been shown to reduce the risk of pyelonephritis.[29] Pregnant women are at increased risk because of anatomical and hormonal changes that contribute to ureteral dilatation and urinary stasis.[28] Typical symptoms of cystitis during pregnancy include dysuria and lower abdominal pain. These symptoms can be associated with fever. Symptoms of pyelonephritis can include flank pain, fever, nausea, vomiting, and costovertebral angle tenderness on examination. Diagnosis is via urinalysis and urine culture.

KEY POINTS

- Urinary tract infection is the most common infection during pregnancy.
- Symptoms include flank pain, fever, nausea, and vomiting.
- Diagnosis is via urinalysis and urine culture.

PELVIC INFLAMMATORY DISEASE

It is rare to have pelvic inflammatory disease or infection of the upper female genital tract during pregnancy. However, this can occur in the first 12 weeks of gestation. The symptoms consist of lower quadrant abdominal pain and fever. Testing consists of a gynecologic examination, examination of vaginal discharge, pregnancy test, CBC, and tests for chlamydia and gonococcus.

KEY POINTS
• Pelvic inflammatory disease most often occurs during the first trimester.
• Symptoms include lower quadrant abdominal pain and fever.
• Diagnosis is via gynecologic examination and testing for chlamydia and gonococcus.

SUMMARY

Abdominal pain can be common during pregnancy. Differentiating whether the pain is pregnancy- or non–pregnancy related is the first step of evaluation. Considering the potential causes of abdominal pain by quadrant can be helpful (Table 4-2). It is important to recognize that the classic presentations of some causes of abdominal pain differ in the gravid state and may not localize to a particular quadrant nor present with fever. As with the evaluation of a nonpregnant patient, a thorough history and physical examination are of utmost importance. Initial laboratory and radiologic evaluation often includes CBC, liver function tests, lipase, urinalysis, and abdominal ultrasound. It is important to keep in mind that pregnancy can influence not only the physical exam findings, but also laboratory findings (Table 4-3). There are several key points in the work-up of abdominal pain during pregnancy (Table 4-4). Perhaps most importantly, the diagnostic evaluation of abdominal pain and necessary therapies should not be delayed until after delivery. Appropriate treatment of the mother will benefit the fetus.

Table 4-2

Considerations of Etiologies of Abdominal Pain by Quadrant

- Right upper quadrant: Hepatitis (AFLP, viral, HELLP, hepatic rupture, Budd-Chiari), cholecystitis/cholangitis, pancreatitis, pneumonia
- Left upper quadrant: Splenic rupture/infarct, pancreatitis, gastritis/PUD
- Left lower quadrant: Diverticulitis, pregnancy-related (ectopic pregnancy, etc), PID, inguinal hernia, nephrolithiasis, IBD
- Right lower quadrant: Appendicitis, pregnancy-related (ectopic pregnancy, etc), PID, inguinal hernia, nephrolithiasis, IBD
- Periumbilical: Early appendicitis, bowel obstruction, pregnancy-related (ectopic pregnancy, etc)
- Epigastric: PUD/gastritis, GERD, pancreatitis, appendicitis, nephrolithiasis, IBD
- Any category: IBS, metabolic causes, peritonitis, toxins (lead poisoning), vascular causes

AFLP: acute fatty liver of pregnancy; HELLP: hemolysis, elevated liver enzymes and low platelets.

Table 4-3

Key Differences in the Evaluation of Abdominal Pain Associated With Pregnancy

- Physical exam findings less reliable
    - ∞ Guarding may not occur related to loss of elasticity of the abdominal wall
    - ∞ Displacement of other abdominal organs by enlarging gravid uterus
- Localization of pain less reliable
- Laboratory evaluations differ with pregnancy
    - ∞ Elevations
        - – WBC count
        - – Alk phos 3- to 4-fold
        - – Ceruloplasmin
        - – Transferrin

(continued)

Table 4-3 *(continued)*

Key Differences in the Evaluation of Abdominal Pain Associated With Pregnancy

> - Amylase
> - D-dimer
> - ESR, CRP, C3, and C4
> - Clotting factors
> ∞ Decreases
>   - Hematocrit
>   - Platelets
>   - Uric acid
>   - Albumin/total protein
> • Choice of radiologic testing can be altered related to radiation exposure
>   ∞ Ultrasound often the first test of choice
>   ∞ MRI can be used in pregnancy, although gadolinium crosses the placental circulation
>   ∞ CT can be used if indicated, but in general is avoided related to fetal radiation exposure

Table 4-4

Key Points: Abdominal Pain and Pregnancy

> • Abdominal pain has a broad differential diagnosis in pregnancy.
>   ∞ Pregnancy-related causes
>   ∞ Non–pregnancy-related causes
> • Thorough history and physical examination is the first step.
>   ∞ Presentations of many causes of abdominal pain differ during pregnancy.
> • Initial laboratory evaluation can include CBC with differential, urinalysis, and tests of liver and pancreatic function.
> • Initial radiologic evaluation can include abdominal ultrasound.
> • Appropriate diagnostic evaluation and therapy should not be delayed until after delivery.
> • Proper treatment of the mother will benefit the fetus.

REFERENCES

1. Wald A, Van Thiel DH, Hoechstetter L, et al. Effect of pregnancy on gastro-intestinal transit. *Dig Dis Sci*. 1982;27(11):1015-1018.
2. Lawson M, Kern F Jr, Everson GT. Gastrointestinal transit time in human pregnancy: prolongation in the second and third trimesters followed by post-partum normalization. *Gastroenterology*. 1985;89(5):996-999.
3. Mintz MC, Grumbach K, Arger PH, Coleman BG. Sonographic evaluation of bile duct size during pregnancy. *AJR Am J Roentgenol*. 1985;145(3):575-578.
4. Woodfield CA, Lazarus E, Chen KC, Mayo-Smith WW. Abdominal pain in pregnancy: diagnoses and imaging unique to pregnancy—review. *AJR Am J Roentgenol*. 2010;194(6, suppl):WS14-WS30.
5. From the Centers for Disease Control and Prevention. Ectopic pregnancy—United States, 1990-1992. *JAMA*. 1995;273(7):533.
6. Tamir IL, Bongard FS, Klein SR. Acute appendicitis in the pregnant patient. *Am J Surg*. 1990;160(6):571-575; discussion 575-576.
7. *Pregnancy in Gastrointestinal Disorders*. Bethesda, MD: American College of Gastroenterology. URL: http://s3.gi.org/physicians/PregnancyMonograph.pdf. Accessed Dec 1, 2011.
8. Hodjati H, Kazerooni T. Location of the appendix in the gravid patient: a re-evaluation of the established concept. *Int J Gynaecol Obstet*. 2003;81(3):245-247.
9. Cappell MS, Colon VJ, Sidhom OA. A study at 10 medical centers of the safety and efficacy of 48 flexible sigmoidoscopies and 8 colonoscopies during pregnancy with follow-up of fetal outcome and with comparison to control groups. *Dig Dis Sci*. 1996;41(12):2353-2361.
10. Cappell MS, Fox SR, Gorrepati N. Safety and efficacy of colonoscopy during pregnancy: an analysis of pregnancy outcome in 20 patients. *J Reprod Med*. 2010;55(3-4):115-123.
11. Wong YS, Liu SY, Ng SS, et al. Giant Meckel's diverticulitis: a rare condition complicating pregnancy. *Am J Surg*. 2010;200(1):184-185.
12. Huerta S, Barleben A, Peck MA, Gordon IL. Meckel's diverticulitis: a rare etiology of an acute abdomen during pregnancy. *Curr Surg*. 2006;63(4):290-293.
13. Thukral C, Wolf JL. Therapy insight: drugs for gastrointestinal disorders in pregnant women. *Nat Clin Pract Gastroenterol Hepatol*. 2006;3(5):256-266.
14. Richter JE. Gastroesophageal reflux disease during pregnancy. *Gastroenterol Clin North Am*. 2003;32(1):235-261.
15. Van Thiel DH, Gavaler JS, Joshi SN, Sara RK, Stremple J. Heartburn of pregnancy. *Gastroenterology*. 1977;72(4, pt 1):666-668.
16. Bruno M. Irritable bowel syndrome and inflammatory bowel disease in pregnancy. *J Perinat Neonatal Nurs*. 2004;18(4):341-350; quiz 351-352.
17. Hasler WL. The irritable bowel syndrome during pregnancy. *Gastroenterol Clin North Am*. 2003;32(1):385-406, viii.
18. Drossman DA. *Rome III: The Functional Gastrointestinal Disorders*. McLean, VA: Degnon Associates Inc; 2006.
19. Stothers L, Lee LM. Renal colic in pregnancy. *J Urol*. 1992;148(5):1383-1387.
20. Marik PE. Venous thromboembolism in pregnancy. *Clin Chest Med*. 2010;31(4):731-740.

21. Heit JA, Kobbervig CE, James AH, Petterson TM, Bailey KR, Melton LJ III. Trends in the incidence of venous thromboembolism during pregnancy or postpartum: a 30-year population-based study. *Ann Intern Med.* 2005;143(10):697-706.

22. Marik PE, Plante LA. Venous thromboembolic disease and pregnancy. *N Engl J Med.* 2008;359(19):2025-2033.

23. Cappell MS, Friedel D. Abdominal pain during pregnancy. *Gastroenterol Clin North Am.* 2003;32(1):1-58.

24. Schmeler KM, Mayo-Smith WW, Peipert JF, Weitzen S, Manuel MD, Gordinier ME. Adnexal masses in pregnancy: surgery compared with observation. *Obstet Gynecol.* 2005;105(5, pt 1):1098-1103.

25. Eyvazzadeh AD, Levine D. Imaging of pelvic pain in the first trimester of pregnancy. *Radiol Clin North Am.* 2006;44(6):863-877.

26. Lim WS, Macfarlane JT, Colthorpe CL. Pneumonia and pregnancy. *Thorax.* 2001;56(5):398-405.

27. Munn MB, Groome LJ, Atterbury JL, Baker SL, Hoff C. Pneumonia as a complication of pregnancy. *J Matern Fetal Med.* 1999;8(4):151-154.

28. Le J, Briggs GG, McKeown A, Bustillo G. Urinary tract infections during pregnancy. *Ann Pharmacother.* 2004;38(10):1692-1701.

29. Schnarr J, Smaill F. Asymptomatic bacteriuria and symptomatic urinary tract infections in pregnancy. *Eur J Clin Invest.* 2008;38(suppl 2):50-57.

5

Constipation in Pregnancy

Yolanda V. Scarlett, MD; Kim L. Isaacs, MD, PhD; and
Millie D. Long, MD, MPH

Constipation is a common gastrointestinal disorder with a reported prevalence of up to 27% in the general population.[1-4] The definition of constipation is symptom-based and may include infrequent bowel movements, incomplete evacuation, straining with defecation, lumpy or hard stools, and a sensation of obstruction or blockage of the anus or rectum with passage of stool.

KEY POINTS
• Constipation's definition is symptom-based.
• Symptoms include the following:
∞ Infrequent bowel movements
∞ Incomplete evacuation
∞ Straining with defecation
∞ Lumpy or hard stools

The Rome III consensus criteria for constipation include 2 or more of the following symptoms: straining during at least 25% of defecations with lumpy or hard stools in at least 25% of defecations

Isaacs KL, Long MD.
GI and Liver Disease During Pregnancy:
A Practical Approach (pp. 61-74).
© 2013 Taylor & Francis Group

Table 5-1

Etiologies of Constipation in Pregnancy

- Decreased fluid intake
- Decreased fiber consumption
- Decreased physical activity
- Metabolic disorders
    - ∞ Thyroid disease
    - ∞ Diabetes mellitus
- Hormonal changes
    - ∞ Increased progesterone
    - ∞ Increased estrogen
    - ∞ Decreased motilin
- Decreased small-bowel motility
- Increased colonic transit time
- Muscular relaxation of the colon
- Pelvic floor dysfunction

or sensation of anorectal obstruction/blockage for at least 25% of defecations; manual maneuvers to facilitate at least 25% of defecations, or fewer than three defecations per week along with rare loose stools; and insufficient criteria for diagnosis of irritable bowel syndrome.[5] Women report symptoms of constipation more frequently than men, and constipation occurring during pregnancy is not uncommon. In the pregnant population, women report straining with defecation, lumpy or hard stools, and sensation of incomplete evacuation more frequently than infrequent bowel movements.[6]

ETIOLOGY

Constipation during pregnancy occurs frequently, and reports range between 11% to 38% in up to more than 50% of pregnant women.[7-9] There are multiple etiologies of constipation in pregnancy, some of which are unique to the gravid female (Table 5-1). As in the general population, pregnant women may have lifestyle modifications contributing to constipation, such as decreased fluid intake, low consumption of fiber, and limited physical activity. In addition, pregnant women may have metabolic factors contributing to constipation, such as diabetes mellitus and thyroid disease.

Several physiologic changes occur during pregnancy that predispose to constipation, including decreased small-bowel motility, prolonged colonic transit time, and muscular relaxation of the colon.[10,11] These changes are attributed to hormonal changes, including increased plasma levels of progesterone, increased estrogen, increased aldosterone levels, and decreased motilin. Progesterone has been demonstrated to have inhibitory effects on both the circular and longitudinal layers of muscle in the colon.[12] In addition, progesterone and estrogen increase renin secretion, which increases aldosterone production via the angiotensin pathway. Increased aldosterone causes increased colonic water absorption, thus increasing risk of constipation.[12]

As pregnancy progresses, the enlarging uterus causes the visceral organs to rearrange and may cause symptoms of constipation.[10] Pregnant women may also experience pelvic floor dysfunction that hampers expulsion of stool, thus contributing to symptoms of constipation. It is important to evaluate and manage constipation, as excessive straining with defecation has been reported to contribute to pudendal nerve injury and pelvic organ prolapse.[13,14]

KEY POINTS

• Constipation is common in pregnancy.
  ∞ Seen in up to 50% of women
• Risk factors
  ∞ Lifestyle: Low fluid intake, low fiber intake, sedentary lifestyle
  ∞ Endocrine: Diabetes and thyroid disease
  ∞ Hormonal changes: Increased progesterone, estrogen, and aldosterone; decreased motilin
  ∞ Mechanical effects of enlarging uterus

WORK-UP OF CONSTIPATION IN THE PREGNANT PATIENT

Work-up of the pregnant woman with constipation is similar to that of the nonpregnant individual. History is very important and will help direct the diagnostic evaluation. The first step is to establish the patient's baseline bowel movement pattern prior to pregnancy and whether it has changed during the course of the pregnancy. The characteristics of the bowel movement pattern, such as frequency, straining, and a sense of incomplete evacuation, may help distinguish between slow transit and obstructive defecation. Likewise, physical description of the stool is often helpful. Hard stool is commonly seen with motility difficulties, whereas soft stool that is difficult to pass may be associated with obstructive difficulties, such as pelvic floor dyssynergia and compression by the gravid uterus.

KEY POINTS

• What are the characteristics of the stool?
  ∞ Is it hard or soft?
  ∞ Is it lumpy?
  ∞ Is it small caliber?

In the nonpregnant patient, radiographic evaluation with sitz markers will help to distinguish between slow transit and obstructive constipation. Due to the radiation risk of an abdominal x-ray, this cannot be performed during pregnancy. Anal manometric and sensation evaluations can be done safely during pregnancy and may help diagnose pudendal nerve injury.[15] Formal rectal manometry should be avoided later in pregnancy due to the theoretic risk of induction of uterine contractions. Likewise, defecography, which may help with diagnosis of a rectocele and pelvic floor abnormalities, involves radiation and is reserved for postpartum diagnostic evaluation. Sigmoidoscopy can be safely performed during pregnancy when indicated and should be used in the diagnostic evaluation if there is a concern for a distal obstruction (see Chapter 8). Most constipation during pregnancy will be due to slow transit rather than obstruction. Laboratory evaluation should include electrolytes, calcium, thyroid-stimulating hormone (TSH), glucose, and CBC.

KEY POINTS

• What are the characteristics of the bowel pattern?
  ∞ Are there fewer than 3 bowel movements per week?
  ∞ Is there straining with 25% or more of bowel movements?
  ∞ Is there a sense of incomplete evacuation with 25% or more of bowel movements?

KEY POINTS
• Laboratory evaluation ∞ Electrolytes, calcium, TSH, glucose, CBC • Diagnostic testing ∞ Look at the stool ∞ Avoid procedures that require radiation: sitz mark study and defecography ∞ Sigmoidoscopy if suspicion is high for distal obstructing mass ∞ Delay manometric testing until after delivery

MANAGEMENT OF CONSTIPATION IN THE PREGNANT PATIENT

The management of constipation in the pregnant woman is similar to that of the nonpregnant woman. An initial assessment should include taking a comprehensive history with inventory of the amount of the fluid and fiber intake along with an assessment of physical activity. Dietary modification should include drinking a minimum of 64 oz of water daily and gradually increasing fiber intake to 20 to 35 g daily. Lifestyle modification of increasing physical activity is recommended if not contraindicated by complications of the pregnancy. Light physical exercise has been shown to be beneficial treatment of constipation in pregnancy.[16] Medications are added to the treatment regimen of constipation in pregnancy if dietary and lifestyle modifications do not provide adequate symptomatic relief. As with any medication prescribed during pregnancy, laxatives need to be assessed for efficacy, safety, and teratogenic potential.

Medications felt safe to use during pregnancy for constipation include psyllium, methylcellulose, polyethylene glycol (PEG), lactulose, senna, bisacodyl, and docusate (Table 5-2). Psyllium and methylcellulose are bulk laxatives, and neither has been classified by the FDA. PEG is an osmotic agent available for daily dosing as brand name MiraLAX (Merck & Co, Inc, Whitehouse Station, NJ). MiraLAX is a Category C drug for pregnancy and has been suggested as the first laxative to try when bulking agents have failed.[17] Lactulose is also an osmotic agent categorized as Category B for use in pregnancy, but its use may be limited by the side effect

Table 5-2

Medication Recommendations for Constipation and Hemorrhoids in Pregnancy and Breastfeeding

	FDA Pregnancy Category*	Pregnancy Comment	Breastfeeding Comment
Constipation			
Magnesium citrate	B	Low risk in short term, avoid long-term use due to electrolyte abnormalities	Compatible
Sodium phosphate	C	Avoid long-term use due to electrolyte abnormalities	Unknown
PEG	C	Compatible	Low risk
Senna	C	Low risk in short term	Compatible
Docusate	C	Low risk	Compatible
Bisacodyl	B	Low risk in short term, can have cramping	Unknown
Lactulose	B	Low risk in short term, can have cramping and bloating	Probably compatible
Castor oil	X	Avoid, uterine contraction and rupture	Possibly unsafe
Mineral oil	C	Avoid, can impair maternal fat-soluble vitamin absorption, neonatal coagulopathy and hemorrhage	Possibly unsafe
Psyllium	Not classified	Low risk	Compatible

(continued)

Table 5-2 *(continued)*

Medication Recommendations for Constipation and Hemorrhoids in Pregnancy and Breastfeeding

	FDA Pregnancy Category*	Pregnancy Comment	Breastfeeding Comment
Methylcellulose	Not classified	Low risk	Compatible
Lubiprostone	C	Avoid, no increased birth defects seen, but studies in guinea pigs show increased risk of miscarriages	Unknown
Hydrocortisone rectal	C	Probably low risk related to low systemic absorption	Unknown
Analpram (hydrocortisone/pramoxine)	C	Probably low risk related to low systemic absorption	Unknown
Proctofoam	C	Probably low risk related to low systemic absorption	Unknown

Adapted from Mahadevan U, Kane S. American gastroenterological association institute medical position statement on the use of gastrointestinal medications in pregnancy. *Gastroenterology.* 2006;131(1):278-282.

*See Appendix for discussion of FDA pregnancy categories.

of abdominal bloating. Senna is a Category C stimulant agent. A recent prospective, controlled study has shown that senna has no teratogenic potential.[18] Bisacodyl is a Category B stimulant laxative that may have limited use secondary to abdominal cramping. Docusate is a Category C emollient agent with limited efficacy. Both mineral oil and castor oil are emollient laxatives. Mineral oil has been associated with malabsorption of fat-soluble vitamins, and castor oil can cause severe abdominal cramping and premature uterine contractions. Both should be avoided during pregnancy. Often, medications can be used in combination as well. For example, MiraLAX combined with docusate, or a short course of a stimulant laxative such as bisacodyl.

Tegaserod, a 5-HT$_4$ agonist prokinetic laxative, classified as a Category B drug, was removed from the market in 2007 and was made available only through restricted distribution through the manufacturer. In April 2008, tegaserod's limited distribution program was suspended by the FDA secondary to ischemic cardiac and cerebral events. Tegaserod is now available upon FDA review only for life-threatening emergency situations or situations requiring hospitalization.[19] Lubiprostone, a chloride channel activator, is classified as a Category C drug. Animal studies have demonstrated no teratogenic effects in rats or rabbits, but lubiprostone has not been studied in human pregnancy.

HEMORRHOIDS

Hemorrhoids are swollen veins at or near the anus. Internal hemorrhoids arise above the dentate line, while external hemorrhoids arise below the dentate line. Normally, hemorrhoids are asymptomatic. However, pregnancy predisposes to symptomatic hemorrhoids. Multiple factors have been associated with the development of hemorrhoids, including straining, chronic constipation, vascular engorgement from increased intra-abdominal pressure, and the absence of valves in hemorrhoidal vessels and draining veins. One reason hemorrhoids may become more symptomatic during pregnancy is that the circulating blood volume increases by 25% to 40%.[20] This increased volume can increase venous dilation and engorgement. Additionally, the enlarging uterus can increase venous stasis. Hemorrhoids are one of the most common anorectal diseases during pregnancy. It has been estimated that 25% to 35% of pregnant women are affected by hemorrhoids.[21,22] By the third trimester, some studies have shown the prevalence of hemorrhoids to be up to 85%.[23] The predominant symptoms of hemorrhoids include intermittent bleeding, burning, and pruritus.

KEY POINTS

- Hemorrhoids are swollen veins at or near the anus.
- Causes include constipation, straining, and increased intra-abdominal pressure.
- They are exacerbated by pregnancy through increasing circulating blood volume and venous stasis from the enlarging uterus.
- Symptoms include intermittent bleeding, burning, and pruritus.

DIAGNOSIS OF HEMORRHOIDS

Because many medical conditions present with rectal bleeding, it is important to evaluate for risk factors for other causes. For example, in a patient with significant diarrhea and rectal bleeding, the differential includes infectious and inflammatory causes of bleeding. Rectal bleeding is also often the sentinel presentation of rectal carcinoma, which can occur in women of childbearing ages. Therefore, a careful history and physical examination should be performed to exclude other causes of rectal bleeding and other red flags that warrant further work-up. For example, rectal bleeding associated with weight loss, fever, diarrhea, abdominal distension, or significant problems with evacuation of stool all warrant further work-up. Anoscopy can be performed at bedside to confirm the diagnosis of hemorrhoids.[23] If hemorrhoids fail to respond to conventional therapies, endoscopic evaluation can be considered to confirm the diagnosis and rule out other colorectal pathology (see Chapter 8).

KEY POINTS

- Careful history and physical examination
- Findings that warrant further work-up when associated with rectal bleeding: Weight loss, fever, diarrhea, abdominal distension, significant problems with stool evacuation
- Anoscopy can be performed at bedside for diagnosis
- Further work-up warranted if hemorrhoids do not respond to conventional therapies

---

TREATMENT OF HEMORRHOIDS

Treatment during pregnancy is directed toward dietary changes to improve constipation, a known exacerbating factor of hemorrhoids, and topical relief of pain. All of the medications and dietary changes used for constipation can be beneficial with hemorrhoids as well. For example, fiber has a beneficial effect in the treatment of symptomatic hemorrhoids. Reducing iron supplementation or changing to slow-release iron can also be of benefit, as iron is associated with increased constipation. Decreased straining during bowel movements shrinks internal hemorrhoidal veins, which can reduce symptoms. A first-line local treatment for hemorrhoids, if dietary measures are not of benefit, is a sitz bath. The warm water of a sitz bath (40° C to 50° C for 10 min) can often relieve anorectal pain.[24] Topical medications including suppositories and ointments that contain local pain medications (benzocaine, dibucaine, or pramoxine), mild astringents (witch hazel), or corticosteroids are also available for the treatment of hemorrhoids. Rectal products containing epinephrine or phenylephrine, which contract blood vessels to reduce hemorrhoidal swelling, should be used with caution during pregnancy.[20] Available topical therapies provide short-term relief from discomfort, pain, and bleeding. Because of the small doses and limited systemic absorption, they can be used by pregnant women; however, not all of these medications have been specifically studied in pregnant women. Hydrocortisone/pramoxine topical therapies (hydrocortisone suppositories, Proctofoam [Schwarz Pharma, Seymour, IN], Analpram [Ferndale Healthcare, Ferndale, MI]) are pregnancy Category C agents,[25,26] with unknown effects on lactation. For many women, symptoms will resolve spontaneously soon after birth, and any corrective treatment (including consideration of surgical therapies) should be deferred until after birth, if possible.

Available office-based procedures for hemorrhoids (which should be deferred during pregnancy, if possible) include band ligation and injection sclerotherapy. Injection sclerotherapy has been found to be safe and effective during pregnancy.[27] Laser coagulation is safe and effective in nonpregnant patients with hemorrhoids and is theoretically safe in pregnant women, although it has not been studied in this population.[20,27] Surgical hemorrhoidectomy is reserved for internal hemorrhoids that prolapse and incarcerate or that fail to respond to office-based procedures. Closed excisional hemorrhoidectomy using local anesthesia has been reported to be safe during pregnancy.[28]

KEY POINTS
• Dietary changes including increased fiber intake
• Avoidance of straining at defecation
• Medical management of constipation
• Change to slow-release iron supplementation
• Sitz baths
• Topical therapies (local pain medications/astringents/corticosteroids)
• Defer corrective treatment (surgery, etc) until after birth if possible

SUMMARY

Overall, constipation and hemorrhoids can be safely managed during pregnancy. Successful management of constipation can improve quality of life for the pregnant woman and may also decrease the risk of damage to the pelvic floor that may increase the risk of chronic constipation. Often, dietary changes, treatment of constipation, and symptomatic therapies such as sitz baths can effectively treat hemorrhoids during pregnancy without further invasive therapies.

REFERENCES

1. Everhart J, Go V, Johannes R, Fitzsimmons S, Toth H, White L. A longitudinal survey of self-reported bowel habits in the United States. *Dig Dis Sci.* 1989;34(8):1153-1162.
2. Drossman D, Li Z, Andruzzi E, et al. U.S. householder survey of functional gastrointestinal disorders: prevalence, sociodemography and health impact. *Dig Dis Sci.* 1993;38(9):1569-1580.
3. Thompson W, Irvine E, Pare P, Ferazzi S, Rance L. Functional gastrointestinal disorders in Canada: first population-based survey using the Rome II criteria with suggestions for improving the questionnaire. *Dig Dis Sci.* 2002;47(1):225-235.
4. Pare P, Ferazzi S, Thompson W, Irvine E, Rance L. An epidemiological survey of constipation in Canada: definitions, rates, demographics and predictors of health care. *Am J Gastroenterol.* 2004;99:750-759.
5. Longstreth G, Thompson W, Chey W, Houghton L, Mearin F, Spiller R. Functional bowel disorders. *Gastroenterology.* 2006;130(5):1480-1491.

6. Bradley CS, Kennedy CM, Turcea AM, Rao SS, Nygaard I. Constipation in pregnancy: prevalence, symptoms, and risk factors. *Obstet Gynecol.* 2007;110(6):1351-1357.

7. Welsh A. Hyperemesis, gastrointestinal and liver disorders in pregnancy. *Curr Obstet Gynaecol.* 2005;15:123-131.

8. Fagan E. *Disorders of the Gastrointestinal Tract.* Boston, MA: Blackwell Publishers; 2002.

9. Gartland D, Brown S, Donath S, Perlen S. Women's health in early pregnancy: findings from an Australian nulliparous cohort study. *Aust N Z J Obstet Gynaecol.* 2010;50(5):413-418.

10. Wald A, Van Thiel DH, Hoechstetter L, et al. Effect of pregnancy on gastrointestinal transit. *Dig Dis Sci.* 1982;27(11):1015-1018.

11. Saha S, Manlolo J, McGowan CE, Reinert S, Degli Esposti S. Gastroenterology consultations in pregnancy. *J Womens Health (Larchmt).* 2011;20(3):359-363.

12. Cullen G, O'Donoghue D. Constipation and pregnancy. *Best Pract Res Clin Gastroenterol.* 2007;21(5):807-818.

13. Spence-Jones C, Kamm MA, Henry MM, Hudson CN. Bowel dysfunction: a pathogenic factor in uterovaginal prolapse and urinary stress incontinence. *Br J Obstet Gynaecol.* 1994;101(2):147-152.

14. Snooks SJ, Barnes PR, Swash M, Henry MM. Damage to the innervation of the pelvic floor musculature in chronic constipation. *Gastroenterology.* 1985;89(5):977-981.

15. Chaliha C, Sultan AH, Bland JM, Monga AK, Stanton SL. Anal function: effect of pregnancy and delivery. *Am J Obstet Gynecology.* 2001;185(2):427-432.

16. Artal R, O'Toole M. Guidelines of the American College of Obstetricians and Gynecologists for exercise during pregnancy and the postpartum period. *Br J Sports Med.* 2003;37(1):6-12.

17. Mahadevan U, Kane S. American gastroenterological association institute technical review on the use of gastrointestinal medications in pregnancy. *Gastroenterology.* 2006;131(1):283-311.

18. Acs N, Bánhidy F, Puhó EH, Czeizel AE. No association between severe constipation with related drug treatment in pregnant women and congenital abnormalities in their offspring: a population-based case-control study. *Congenit Anom (Kyoto).* 2010;50(1):15-20.

19. Thompson CA. News. Novartis suspends tegaserod sales at FDA's request. *Am J Health Syst Pharm.* 2007;64(10):1020.

20. Wald A. Constipation, diarrhea, and symptomatic hemorrhoids during pregnancy. *Gastroenterol Clin North Am.* 2003;32(1):309-322, vii.

21. Staroselsky A, Nava-Ocampo AA, Vohra S, Koren G. Hemorrhoids in pregnancy. *Can Fam Physician.* 2008;54(2):189-190.

22. Abramowitz L, Sobhani I, Benifla JL, et al. Anal fissure and thrombosed external hemorrhoids before and after delivery. *Dis Colon Rectum.* 2002;45(5):650-655.

23. Gojnic M, Dugalic V, Papic M, Vidakovic S, Milicevic S, Pervulov M. The significance of detailed examination of hemorrhoids during pregnancy. *Clin Exp Obstet Gynecol.* 2005;32(3):183-184.

24. Shafik A. Role of warm-water bath in anorectal conditions. The "thermosphincteric reflex." *J Clin Gastroenterol.* 1993;16(4):304-308.

25. Vohra S, Akoury H, Bernstein P, et al. The effectiveness of Proctofoam-HC for treatment of hemorrhoids in late pregnancy. *J Obstet Gynaecol Can.* 2009;31(7):654-659.

26. Ebrahimi N, Vohra S, Gedeon C, et al. The fetal safety of hydrocortisone-pramoxine (Proctofoam-HC) for the treatment of hemorrhoids in late pregnancy. *J Obstet Gynaecol Can.* 2011;33(2):153-158.

27. Medich DS, Fazio VW. Hemorrhoids, anal fissure, and carcinoma of the colon, rectum, and anus during pregnancy. *Surg Clin North Am.* 1995; 75(1):77-88.

28. Saleeby RG Jr, Rosen L, Stasik JJ, Riether RD, Sheets J, Khubchandani IT. Hemorrhoidectomy during pregnancy: risk or relief? *Dis Colon Rectum.* 1991;34(3):260-261.

6

Irritable Bowel Syndrome

Millie D. Long, MD, MPH and
Spencer D. Dorn, MD, MPH

Irritable bowel syndrome (IBS) is characterized by altered bowel habits and abdominal pain. IBS is extremely common. It affects up to 20% of the general population[1] and is the most common diagnosis in outpatient gastroenterology clinics.[2] Notably, women are affected up to 2 to 3 times more often than men,[1] and IBS often develops at a young age, typically coinciding with the childbearing years. Therefore, recognizing and treating symptoms of IBS prior to and during pregnancy becomes important. The Rome III criteria for diagnosis of IBS are listed in Table 6-1. In brief, IBS is characterized by recurrent abdominal pain or discomfort that improves upon defecation and/or is associated with a change in stool frequency or consistency.[3]

While no large studies of IBS during pregnancy exist, bowel habits often change during pregnancy: 11% to 38% of pregnant women report constipation, and approximately one-third report increased stool frequency.[4-7] Risk factors for constipation during pregnancy include iron supplementation and past constipation treatment.[7] In a prospective study of gastrointestinal (GI) conditions in pregnancy,

Isaacs KL, Long MD.
GI and Liver Disease During Pregnancy:
A Practical Approach (pp. 75-90).
© 2013 Taylor & Francis Group

Table 6-1

Rome III Criteria for Diagnosis of IBS

- Recurrent abdominal pain or discomfort at least 3 days/month over the past 3 months
- Pain associated with at least 2 of the following:
  - ∞ Improvement with defecation
  - ∞ Onset with a change in frequency of stool
  - ∞ Onset with a change in appearance of stool

an IBS diagnosis (by Rome II criteria) was found in 19%, 13%, and 13% of pregnant women in the first, second, and third trimesters, respectively.[7]

SYMPTOMS

Predominant stool consistency can be measured through the Bristol stool scale.[8] This scale describes 7 total types of stool, ranging from types indicating constipation to types indicating diarrhea. The first type is hard lumps of stool that are hard to pass, similar to nuts. Type 2 refers to sausage-shaped, lumpy stool. Type 3 is like a sausage, but with cracks on the surface. Type 4 is like a sausage or snake, but smooth and soft. Type 5 refers to easily passed soft blobs of stool, with clear-cut edges. Type 6 is fluffy pieces of stool with ragged edges that are mushy. Type 7 is entirely liquid stool without solid pieces. This scale is used to sub-divide IBS into one of 4 sub-types: IBS with constipation (IBS-C), IBS with diarrhea (IBS-D), IBS-mixed (IBS-M), or IBS-Unclassified (IBS-U). Those with IBS-C frequently pass hard stools, whereas those with IBS-D frequently pass loose stools. Those with IBS-M have both hard and loose stools within hours or days, whereas those with IBS-U infrequently have either. The characteristics of IBS sub-types by Bristol scale are shown in Figure 6-1.

Like stool pattern, abdominal discomfort (the hallmark IBS symptom) also varies widely. Some experience abdominal pain, which can vary in location, intensity, and triggering factors. Others experience bloating, which is one of the most bothersome IBS symptoms.[9] Additionally, IBS frequently co-occurs with upper GI symptoms (eg, nausea, heartburn) as well as non-GI

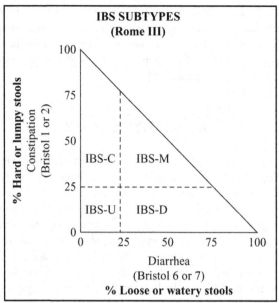

Figure 6-1. Characteristics of IBS Sub-types by Bristol Scale. (Reprinted with permission from Drossman DA. Rome III: *The functional gastrointestinal disorders.* McLean, VA: Degnon Associates, Inc; 2006.)

symptoms (eg, headaches, back pain). One particular challenge is that pregnancy is associated with changes in bowel habits, abdominal discomfort, upper GI symptoms, and even non-GI symptoms. With this constellation of common symptoms, differentiation of etiologies (including IBS) can be difficult.

ASSOCIATED FACTORS

Psychosocial stressors often play a role in IBS and sometimes occur prior to the onset of bowel symptoms. For instance, Drossman and colleagues showed that sexual abuse is a risk factor for IBS.[10] Likewise, patients with IBS are more likely to have abnormal personality patterns and display greater illness behaviors than the general population.[11] Other possible contributing factors, including imbalances in the GI bacterial flora ("microbiome"),[12] dietary factors (eg, concomitant lactose, fructose, or sorbitol intolerance), and hormonal factors (particularly those associated with the menstrual cycle), can be associated with increased symptoms in women with IBS.[13] It is also possible that the hormonal changes associated with pregnancy can modify IBS symptoms, although this has not been studied specifically in pregnancy.

PATHOPHYSIOLOGY

The pathophysiology of IBS is not entirely understood. However, those with IBS are characterized by visceral hypersensitivity, intestinal dysmotility, and disturbance of the brain-gut axis. The reasons for these abnormalities are largely unknown, although they have been linked to genetic factors, early childhood learning, emotional trauma, GI infection, microscopic inflammation, abnormal autonomic nervous system function, hormonal changes, psychological factors, dietary factors, and disturbed microbial flora.[4] Considering these disparate factors, IBS may be best explained by the biopsychosocial model, in which genetic, environmental, psychological, and physiologic factors contribute to IBS development and outcomes.

DIAGNOSIS

Diagnosing IBS can be challenging. Because there is no biomarker, physicians must rely on symptoms, which tend to vary between and even among individuals and can sometimes be caused by "organic" GI diseases. Consequently, clinicians often consider IBS a "diagnosis of exclusion" that can only be made after a series of diagnostic tests are negative. However, in those who satisfy the Rome criteria and do not have any "alarm symptoms" (eg, hematochezia, weight loss, nocturnal symptoms, fever, or family history of colon cancer or inflammatory bowel disease), diagnostic testing is low yield. Instead, these individuals can be positively diagnosed based on symptoms, history, and physical exam alone.[14] Those with alarm symptoms, or symptoms that progressively worsen despite therapy, may be considered for further testing.

So what about IBS during pregnancy? Certainly, as IBS is a chronic ongoing disorder, those with this diagnosis prior to pregnancy should proceed with therapeutic management during pregnancy rather than further testing. There are no large studies following women with IBS through pregnancy; therefore, it is difficult to know whether their symptoms change or whether modified therapeutic regimens are needed.

KEY POINTS

• The following are alarm symptoms:
  ∞ Bleeding
  ∞ Weight loss
  ∞ Fever
  ∞ Nocturnal awakening with pain and/or diarrhea

For pregnant women who present with new-onset symptoms (eg, alteration of bowel pattern and abdominal discomfort), the first step is a detailed history and physical exam. Any new medication or supplements should be noted, as many can be associated with diarrhea and/or constipation. Duration of symptoms is important, as is the nature of onset. Basic laboratory evaluation in the pregnant woman with new-onset of IBS symptoms (abdominal discomfort, diarrhea, and/or constipation) is also warranted, including CBC, electrolytes, and thyroid testing. Alarm symptoms such as hematochezia and/or weight loss may prompt additional testing, including endoscopic evaluation (see Chapters 7 and 8). Further specific history and testing should be obtained based on the predominant symptom, as outlined next.

KEY POINTS

• No further work-up is needed in those with IBS diagnosed prior to pregnancy and characteristic symptoms.
• History and physical examination are the first steps.
• Basic laboratory evaluation can include the following:
  ∞ CBC
  ∞ Electrolytes
  ∞ Thyroid testing
  ∞ Stool studies to rule out infection in those with diarrhea
• Further work-up should be based on the predominant symptom.
• Endoscopic evaluation is not indicated during pregnancy unless alarm symptoms or other abnormal findings present on initial work-up.

WORK-UP BY PREDOMINANT SYMPTOM

In general, in the absence of red flag symptoms or abnormal physical exam findings, an extensive diagnostic evaluation is not initially needed. Often, one can start with directed therapy toward the predominant symptom (diarrhea or constipation) for a limited time period (3 to 6 weeks).[4] If there is no response, further diagnostic work-up may then be indicated.

CONSTIPATION

Work-up of constipation in the absence of red flag symptoms or abnormal physical exam findings is not indicated. Studies such as radiologic evaluation with sitz markers to document colonic inertia or anorectal manometry to assess for pelvic floor dyssynergia should be delayed until after delivery (see Chapter 5). Dietary and medical therapies should be employed to treat constipation symptomatically.

KEY POINTS
• Perform history and physical with basic evaluation.   • Treat symptomatically unless there are red flags or abnormal laboratory or examination findings.   • No endoscopic evaluation is needed.

DIARRHEA

Work-up of the pregnant individual with nonbloody diarrhea starts with history. Specific questions should be asked, such as the stool appearance (eg, whether it is bloody, greasy, floats in the toilet bowl, malodorous), overall volume, frequency, including whether there is nocturnal awakening for diarrhea, and symptoms of dehydration. The presence of hematochezia, nocturnal diarrhea, and/or symptoms of dehydration, as well as abnormalities on physical exam should provoke further testing. Initial testing should include stool studies to rule out chronic infection, such as *Clostridium difficile*. Additionally, stool electrolytes (sodium, potassium) can be performed to assess for an osmotic versus secretory diarrhea. It is also reasonable to perform a laxative screening test on the stool when symptoms appear atypical. Stool output should also be quantified in those reporting high-volume or nocturnal diarrhea. The output can also be tested for fat to ensure that there is not a component of malabsorption. If there is an index of suspicion based on risk factors, such as iron deficiency anemia or a family history of celiac disease, serologic testing for celiac disease can be performed (serum tissue transglutaminase [TTG] or anti-endomysial antibody [EMA] levels, with serum IgA level). In those with specific dietary triggers, a lactose breath test can be considered, though a trial of dietary avoidance may be easier. Serum markers of inflammation can also be tested if there is a suspicion for inflammatory bowel disease (IBD), although these markers can be elevated related to pregnancy itself. Endoscopic evaluation should be deferred if possible until after delivery. If endoscopic evaluation is required related to ongoing refractory symptoms, red flag symptoms, or suspicion of new-onset IBD, this should be performed during the second trimester if possible (see Chapter 8).

KEY POINTS

- History and physical with basic evaluation
  - ∞ Characteristics of the stool, volume, and nocturnal awakening
  - ∞ Specific dietary triggers
  - ∞ Signs of inflammatory bowel disease (skin rashes, joint abnormalities, oral ulcerations)
- Further testing if indicated
  - ∞ Infection *(C difficile)*
  - ∞ Stool volume
  - ∞ Stool fat
  - ∞ Stool electrolytes
  - ∞ Celiac testing as appropriate
  - ∞ Breath test for lactose intolerance
  - ∞ Endoscopic evaluation deferred until after delivery unless red flags, severe symptoms, or suspicion of new-onset IBD

PAIN

A general history and physical should be performed, with diagnostic testing as needed based on the location, severity, characterization, and frequency of the pain and whether there are any red flag symptoms. For a complete description of the work-up of abdominal pain, see Chapter 4. For pain meeting the definition of IBS in the Rome III criteria,[3] therapeutic trials based on predominant symptoms should be initiated.

KEY POINTS
• History and physical examination should be performed with the basic evaluation.
• Location, severity, characterization, and frequency guide further work-up.
• If pain meets definition of IBS in Rome Criteria, therapeutic trials based on predominant symptoms can be initiated.

TREATMENT

There is no cure for IBS. Rather, the goal of therapy is to manage symptoms and maximize quality of life. The cornerstone of treatment is a strong provider-patient relationship. It is important to explain IBS and reassure patients that the condition will not shorten their lifespans or affect their developing fetuses. In addition, diet may be changed. Often, we recommend eating smaller, more frequent meals, increasing fiber, and keeping a food diary to recommend possible foods that exacerbate symptoms. Those with significant bloating and diarrhea may improve with a reduction in dietary sugars, such as in the Fermentable Oligo-, Di- and Monosaccharides, and Polyols (FODMAP) diet. Various medications are available. The specific choice often depends on the predominant IBS symptom (see below). Finally, psychologically based therapies can be used to treat IBS. These include cognitive behavioral therapy, hypnosis, relaxation therapy, generalized biofeedback, stress management, and mindfulness meditation.

CONSTIPATION

The first-line therapy for constipation-predominant IBS is increased fiber supplementation. If the individual does not respond to fiber, an osmotic laxative containing polyethylene glycol (PEG) should be used (Category C). In fact, in a consensus conference of the management of constipation during pregnancy, PEG was considered to be an ideal laxative as it is effective, not absorbed, and well tolerated.[15,16] Other classes of osmotic laxatives include saline osmotic (magnesium and sodium salts) and saccharated osmotic (lactulose and sorbitol). Magnesium citrate (Category B) has a rapid onset of action and is only recommended for short-term use to avoid electrolyte disarray. Lactulose is a Category B agent that is an effective laxative, but its use can be limited by cramping and bloating. Stimulant laxatives such as bisacodyl (Category C) and senna (Category C) can be used for short-term relief of symptoms. These agents can be associated with cramping. Docusate, a stool softener, is considered low risk in pregnancy (Category C). Castor oil (Category X) and mineral oil (Category C) are contraindicated, as castor oil can stimulate uterine contractions and mineral oil can impair maternal fat-soluble vitamin absorption.[16]

DIARRHEA

The goals are to add bulk to the stool, slow down transit, and thereby improve the sensation of urgency. Kaopectate (Chattem, Inc, Chattanooga, TN), which contains kaolin and pectin, can add bulk to the stool. However, as this agent now contains bismuth subsalicylate in its formulation, its use is no longer routinely recommended. The salicylates can be absorbed, causing premature closure of ductus arteriosus, complications to the fetus such as hemorrhage or decreased birth weight, and possible teratogenicity.[16] Loperamide can be an effective antidiarrheal agent, but should be used in moderation. This agent is likely safe for use during pregnancy (Category C), although there has been one report of possible cardiovascular defects. Lomotil (atropine/diphenoxylate) is another antidiarrheal agent (Category C) and should be used only in moderation when indicated. Reports of teratogenicity in animals exist. Antispasmodics, such as hyoscyamine (Category C) and dicyclomine (Category B), can slow down colonic transit via their anticholinergic effects. As with other agents, antispasmodics should be used with caution as little to no human data on safety exist. There have been reports of congenital anomalies associated with dicyclomine. Bile acid sequestrants are another class of agents used in diarrhea, and these agents (such as cholestyramine) are pregnancy Category C. Fat-soluble vitamin deficiency, including coagulopathy, can be associated with cholestyramine. These agents are typically used in those with diarrhea due to prior bowel resections or cholecystectomy. While considered low risk, cholestyramine should be used with caution. For those with specific dietary triggers, avoidance of these triggers via dietary manipulation should be considered rather than pharmacologic therapies. Often, individuals can improve diarrhea with a diet low in fat and/or dairy products.

PAIN

Pain in IBS can be difficult to manage. Opiate pain medications should be avoided both for pregnant and nonpregnant individuals. Opiates may only provide temporary relief and can be associated with a significant risk of dependence. Opioids can be associated with significant GI side effects such as reduced motility, nausea, vomiting, constipation, and gastroparesis. Additionally, there can be a risk of narcotic bowel syndrome (NBS). NBS is associated with chronic or recurrent abdominal pain that worsens with continued or escalating dosages of opiates.[17] Often, antidepressants are used in the treatment of pain-predominant IBS. Classes of medications such as the tricyclic antidepressants (TCA), selective serotonin reuptake inhibitors (SSRI), and serotonin norepinephrine reuptake inhibitors (SNRI) are often used in the nonpregnant patient. The TCAs are Pregnancy Category C and D. In general, these agents may be associated with worse outcomes and should likely be avoided during pregnancy. The majority of SSRIs and SNRIs are Category C, with the exception of paroxetine, which is Category D and is related to a higher absolute rate of birth defects when compared to other antidepressants. The safety of antidepressant drugs during pregnancy has been studied for the indication of depression, but not for IBS. Maternal use of SSRIs during early pregnancy is not associated with significantly increased risks of congenital heart defects or of most other categories of birth defects. However, caution should be used with these medications during pregnancy.[18] SSRI and SNRI exposure late in pregnancy can lead to serotonin reuptake inhibitor-related symptoms in up to 30% of exposed infants postnatally. Symptoms are generally mild and self-limited, but infants are often observed for as much as 48 hours, as some infants require intervention.[18] Only limited data are available regarding the long-term neurodevelopmental outcomes after SSRI exposure during pregnancy and lactation. Therefore, initiation of an antidepressant for an IBS indication during pregnancy has not been specifically studied and should be avoided unless indicated from a psychiatric standpoint.

Alternative aspects of care for the pregnant patient with IBS can include psychological support, reassurance, and educational materials to improve coping skills. In refractory cases of pain in IBS, psychological interventions can be considered. In the pregnant patient, this may be a particularly important aspect of IBS treatment. Psychological counseling may have particular benefits among women with concerns about risks of drugs during pregnancy. One form of psychological therapy, cognitive behavioral therapy (CBT), refers to a partnership between the therapist and the patient using both cognitive and behavioral techniques. These techniques teach the patient strategies for dealing with situations in a way that reduces unwanted symptoms. Components of a CBT program could include relaxation techniques, mindfulness training, or even hypnosis. Mindfulness training has been shown to reduce bowel symptom severity, improve health-related quality of life, and reduce distress in women.[19]

SUMMARY

As IBS is a frequent diagnosis among young adult women, symptoms often coincide with child-bearing years. A "positive" diagnosis can be made for patients who meet Rome Criteria for IBS[3] and lack red flag symptoms. For those with alarming symptoms, a directed work-up may be indicated. Once diagnosed, therapy focuses on the doctor-patient relationship with an emphasis on education and reassurance. Dietary changes, psychologically based therapies, and medications based on the predominant symptom may be helpful, though some drugs must be used cautiously during pregnancy (Table 6-2).

Table 6-2

Medication Recommendations for Pregnancy and Breastfeeding in Irritable Bowel Syndrome

	FDA Pregnancy Category*	Pregnancy Comment	Breastfeeding Comment
Constipation			
Magnesium citrate	B	Low risk in short term, avoid long-term use due to electrolyte abnormalities	Compatible
Sodium phosphate	C	Avoid long-term use due to electrolyte abnormalities	Unknown
PEG	C	Compatible	Low risk
Senna	C	Low risk in short term	Compatible
Docusate	C	Low risk	Compatible
Bisacodyl	C	Low risk in short term, can have cramping	Unknown
Lactulose	B	Low risk in short term, can have cramping and bloating	Probably compatible
Castor oil	X	Avoid, uterine contraction and rupture	Possibly unsafe
Mineral oil	C	Avoid, can impair maternal fat-soluble vitamin absorption, neonatal coagulopathy, and hemorrhage	Possibly unsafe

(continued)

Table 6-2 *(continued)*

Medication Recommendations for Pregnancy and Breastfeeding in Irritable Bowel Syndrome

	FDA Pregnancy Category*	Pregnancy Comment	Breastfeeding Comment
Diarrhea			
Kaopectate	C	Avoid, now contains bismuth	Probably compatible
Bismuth subsalicylate	C	Avoid, possible teratogenicity, hemorrhage, decreased birth weight	Potential toxicity
Loperamide	C	Low risk, possible increased cardiovascular anomalies	Probably compatible
Diphenoxylate/ atropine	C	Potential toxicity: teratogenic in animals	Potential toxicity
Dicyclomine	B	Potential toxicity: possible congenital abnormalities	Potential toxicity
Hyoscyamine	C	Unknown	Probably compatible
Cholestyramine	C	Low risk, potential for vitamin malabsorption and coagulopathy	Compatible
Pain			
TCAs (Amitryptyline, Desipramine, Imipramine, Nortriptyline)	C, D	Avoid, no malformations but worse outcomes	Potential toxicity

(continued)

Table 6-2 *(continued)*

Medication Recommendations for Pregnancy and Breastfeeding in Irritable Bowel Syndrome

	FDA Pregnancy Category*	Pregnancy Comment	Breastfeeding Comment
SSRI (except paroxetine)	C	Potential toxicity: risk of serotonin symptoms in infant when used late in pregnancy, no malformations	Potential toxicity
Paroxetine	D	Avoid: increased birth defects when compared to other SSRI	Potential toxicity
SNRI	C	Potential toxicity: risk of serotonin symptoms in infant when used late in pregnancy	Potential toxicity

Adapted from Mahadevan U, Kane S. American Gastroenterological Association Institute medical position statement on the use of gastrointestinal medications in pregnancy. *Gastroenterology.* 2006;131(1):278-282.

*See Appendix for discussion of FDA pregnancy categories.

REFERENCES

1. Saito YA, Schoenfeld P, Locke GR III. The epidemiology of irritable bowel syndrome in North America: a systematic review. *Am J Gastroenterol.* 2002;97(8):1910-1915.
2. Ferguson A, Sircus W, Eastwood MA. Frequency of "functional" GI disorders. *Lancet.* 1977;2(8038):613-614.
3. Drossman DA. *Rome III: The Functional Gastrointestinal Disorders.* McLean, VA: Degnon Associates Inc; 2006.
4. Hasler WL. The irritable bowel syndrome during pregnancy. *Gastroenterol Clin North Am.* 2003;32(1):385-406, viii.
5. Levy N, Lemberg E, Sharf M. Bowel habit in pregnancy. *Digestion.* 1971;4(4):216-222.
6. Greenhalf JO, Leonard HS. Laxatives in the treatment of constipation in pregnant and breast-feeding mothers. *Practitioner.* 1973;210(256):259-263.

7. Bradley CS, Kennedy CM, Turcea AM, Rao SS, Nygaard IE. Constipation in pregnancy: prevalence, symptoms, and risk factors. *Obstet Gynecol.* 2007;110(6):1351-1357.

8. Heaton KW, O'Donnell LJ. An office guide to whole-gut transit time. Patients' recollection of their stool form. *J Clin Gastroenterol.* 1994;19(1):28-30.

9. Quigley EM. Impact of bloating and distention in irritable bowel syndrome: have we wandered too far from the Manning creed? *Clin Gastroenterol Hepatol.* 2009;7(1):7-8.

10. Drossman DA. Irritable bowel syndrome and sexual/physical abuse history. *Eur J Gastroenterol Hepatol.* 1997;9(4):327-330.

11. Drossman DA, McKee DC, Sandler RS, et al. Psychosocial factors in the irritable bowel syndrome. A multivariate study of patients and nonpatients with irritable bowel syndrome. *Gastroenterology.* 1988;95(3):701-708.

12. Ford AC, Spiegel BM, Talley NJ, Moayyedi P. Small intestinal bacterial overgrowth in irritable bowel syndrome: systematic review and meta-analysis. *Clin Gastroenterol Hepatol.* 2009;7(12):1279-1286.

13. Kane SV, Sable K, Hanauer SB. The menstrual cycle and its effect on inflammatory bowel disease and irritable bowel syndrome: a prevalence study. *Am J Gastroenterol.* 1998;93(10):1867-1872.

14. Spiegel BM, Farid M, Esrailian E, Talley J, Chang L. Is irritable bowel syndrome a diagnosis of exclusion?: a survey of primary care providers, gastroenterologists, and IBS experts. *Am J Gastroenterol.* 2010;105(4):848-858.

15. Tytgat GN, Heading RC, Muller-Lissner S, et al. Contemporary understanding and management of reflux and constipation in the general population and pregnancy: a consensus meeting. *Aliment Pharmacol Ther.* 2003;18(3):291-301.

16. Mahadevan U, Kane S. American Gastroenterological Association Institute medical position statement on the use of GI medications in pregnancy. *Gastroenterology.* 2006;131(1):278-282.

17. Grunkemeier DM, Cassara JE, Dalton CB, Drossman DA. The narcotic bowel syndrome: clinical features, pathophysiology, and management. *Clin Gastroenterol Hepatol.* 2007;5(10):1126-1139; quiz 1121-1122.

18. Alwan S, Reefhuis J, Rasmussen SA, Olney RS, Friedman JM. Use of selective serotonin-reuptake inhibitors in pregnancy and the risk of birth defects. *N Engl J Med.* 2007;356(26):2684-2692.

19. Gaylord SA, Palsson OS, Garland EL, et al. Mindfulness training reduces the severity of irritable bowel syndrome in women: results of a randomized controlled trial. *Am J Gastroenterol.* 2011;106(9):1678-1688.

7

Inflammatory Bowel Disease

Lindsay E. Jones, MD and Millie D. Long, MD, MPH

Inflammatory bowel disease (IBD), specifically ulcerative colitis (UC) and Crohn's disease (CD), commonly affects women during their childbearing years, with a peak age of onset between 15 and 30 years of age.[1] Because of this, the effects of pregnancy on IBD and of IBD on pregnancy become important. Approximately 25% of women conceive for the first time after IBD diagnosis.[2] In general, women with IBD have normal pregnancy outcomes, other than a higher risk of impaired fetal growth.[3] They can have an increased risk of maternal complications, such as venous thromboembolism or malnutrition.[4] Often, women with IBD are concerned about fertility, the risk of inheritance of the disorder, disease activity, and the safety of IBD medications during pregnancy.[5] In fact, in a study of women's perceptions of pregnancy and IBD, Mountifield and colleagues found that 84% reported unwarranted concerns about the effect of IBD medications on pregnancy, and the majority had poor awareness of the detrimental effect of IBD exacerbation during pregnancy.[6] As such, issues pertaining to the management and counseling of the pregnant patient with IBD are of prime clinical importance.

Isaacs KL, Long MD.
*GI and Liver Disease During Pregnancy:
A Practical Approach (pp. 91-116).*
© 2013 Taylor & Francis Group

FERTILITY

Fertility, or the ability to conceive within 1 year of unprotected intercourse, is similar to that of normal age-matched controls in women with IBD.[7] The one exception is if women have had pelvic surgery for their disease.[8,9] A history of pelvic surgery increases the likelihood of pelvic adhesions or scarring, which can impair normal tubal function. Infertility, defined as the inability to conceive after 12 consecutive months of unprotected intercourse, increases 3-fold in women with UC after total abdominal colectomy and ileal-pouch anal anastomosis (IPAA). In a recent meta-analysis, the weighted average infertility rate in medically treated UC was 15% (similar to the overall infertility rate in the United States of 13.8%), and the weighted average infertility rate was 48% after IPAA.[9] One proposal for minimizing this risk of infertility is a staged operation, where total abdominal colectomy is performed initially, and reconstruction with IPAA is deferred until after the reproductive years. Other possible risk factors for infertility in patients with IBD include an acute flare of disease, other pelvic surgery, and active inflammation.[10] Inflammation can cause scarring of the ovaries or fallopian tubes, thereby contributing to infertility.

Other associated factors that influence fertility rates in women with IBD can include sexual dysfunction such as dyspareunia,[6,11] disease-related complications from perianal disease, fistulas, or infections, as well as medication side effects from steroids, which can lead to decreased libido.

KEY POINTS
• Fertility in women with IBD is similar to the general population (except in those with prior pelvic surgery).
• A history of pelvic surgery, particularly IPAA formation, can cause a 3-fold increase in infertility.

INHERITANCE: COUNSELING THE PARENTS

There is a higher relative risk of inheritance of CD or UC in the offspring of patients with IBD. However, this risk is multifactorial, and environmental factors also likely play a large role. The risk for the offspring is estimated to be 2 to 13 times higher when a parent has IBD when compared to the general population. The absolute risk for developing IBD is estimated to be 5% if one parent has CD, 1.7% if one parent has UC, and 35% if both parents have IBD.[5,12]

KEY POINTS

- Relative risk of IBD in offspring is elevated by a factor of 2 to 13 when compared to general population.
- Absolute risk of IBD in offspring remains low when one parent is affected (≤5%).

EFFECT OF DISEASE ACTIVITY ON PREGNANCY

The most important factor for a healthy, successful pregnancy in women with IBD is inactive disease. Disease activity at conception has been associated with preterm birth and low birth weight.[13,14] A recent cohort study from the Netherlands demonstrated that active luminal disease prior to pregnancy was associated with an increased risk of pregnancy complications (OR: 2.8; 95% CI: 1.0 to 7.4).[15] There are also some data to suggest that babies born to women with CD, regardless of disease activity, have lower birth weights.[16] Kornfeld and colleagues demonstrated increased odds of low birth weight, preterm delivery, and C-section delivery among a Swedish cohort of women with IBD.[17] A recent community-based study from northern California demonstrated that women with IBD are at an increased risk for a spontaneous abortion (OR: 1.65; 95% CI: 1.09 to 2.48); an adverse pregnancy outcome (stillbirth, preterm birth, or small for gestational age [SGA] infant; OR: 1.54; 95% CI: 1.00 to 2.38); or a complication of labor (OR: 1.78; 95% CI: 1.13 to 2.81).[18] The study did not find a difference in the rate of congenital malformations in children born to women with IBD. A meta-analysis on IBD in pregnancy found similar results. There was a 1.87-fold increase in prematurity (<37 weeks gestation; 95% CI: 1.52 to 2.31; $p < 0.001$) compared with controls. The incidence of low birth weight (<2500 g) was more than twice that of normal controls (95% CI:

1.38 to 3.19; $p < 0.001$). Women with IBD were 1.5 times more likely to undergo C-section (95% CI: 1.26 to 1.79; $p < 0.001$). However, this meta-analysis did find a 2.37-fold (95% CI: 1.47 to 3.82; $p < 0.001$) increased risk of congenital abnormalities.[19] The main goal for a woman attempting to conceive is to achieve remission at least 3 months prior to conception. If a woman achieves and maintains remission prior to pregnancy, there is a reasonable expectation that she should be able to carry a pregnancy to term without complication.

KEY POINTS
• IBD can be associated with preterm birth and low birth weight. • IBD can be associated with complications of labor. • IBD is associated with an increased rate of C-section delivery. • Active luminal IBD prior to pregnancy is associated with increased pregnancy complications. • Ideally, a woman should enter pregnancy in remission.

EFFECTS OF PREGNANCY ON INFLAMMATORY BOWEL DISEASE

Pregnant women with IBD are as likely to flare as nonpregnant women with IBD (approximately 34% per year).[14,20] Some women with autoimmune conditions have reported lower disease activity during pregnancy. An explanation for this phenomenon is the hypothesis that human leukocyte antigen (HLA) class II disparity between the mother and paternal alloantigens in the fetus induces a protective down-regulation of the immune system.[21] A study by Agret and colleagues showed that CD activity is mildly but significantly lower during pregnancy, with a reduction in tobacco consumption possibly being a contributing factor to the observed improvement.[22] A small cohort study also demonstrated lower rates of relapse of IBD in the 3 years postpartum when compared to the antepartum period.[23] The postpartum time period can also be associated with flares of IBD for several reasons. Discontinuation of medications to breastfeed, hormonal shifts, and changes in inflammatory cytokines may all play a role.[5]

KEY POINTS
• Rates of flare during pregnancy do not change (~34%). • Continuation of medications for IBD during and after pregnancy is important.

BREASTFEEDING

Compared with the general population (60%), patients with IBD (44%) or CD alone (29%) have lower reported rates of breastfeeding reported in one study.[24] A second, more recent study from Manitoba showed that women with IBD have comparable rates of breastfeeding to the general population.[25] In some autoimmune conditions, it has been hypothesized that elevated prolactin associated with lactation may be associated with pro-inflammatory properties, including upregulation of tumor necrosis factor (TNF). A prior study by Kane and colleagues did not show breastfeeding to be associated with increased disease activity, independent of medication cessation.[24] Moffatt and colleagues showed a nonsignificant inverse association between breastfeeding and flare of disease in the postpartum period.[25] Therefore, breastfeeding does not necessarily impact IBD course unless it is associated with discontinuation of medications. The decision to breastfeed should therefore be made independently of disease course, recognizing that medications for IBD should be continued in the postpartum period.

KEY POINTS
• Many mothers with IBD breastfeed. • Breastfeeding is not independently associated with worsened disease activity. • If at all possible, medications for IBD should not be discontinued in order to breastfeed.

MEDICAL TREATMENT OF INFLAMMATORY BOWEL DISEASE DURING PREGNANCY

To minimize the risk of complications to the mother and the fetus, every attempt should be made to achieve remission prior to conception and to maintain remission throughout the pregnancy. Despite limited data, most IBD medications are considered low risk during conception, pregnancy, and lactation with the exception of methotrexate and thalidomide, both of which are absolutely contraindicated in pregnancy.[26] The safety of medical therapies for IBD during pregnancy and breastfeeding is shown in Table 7-1.

AMINOSALICYLATES DURING PREGNANCY

Aminosalicylates are considered low risk for use in pregnancy. Most mesalamines, sulfasalazine, and balsalazide are Pregnancy Category B. Recently, the brands Asacol and Asacol HD (Warner Chilcott, LLC, Rockaway, NJ [both brands of mesalamine]) were moved to Category C. This is due to an inactive ingredient in the enteric coating of these specific agents. Dibutyl phthalate (DBP), found in the coating, has been associated with external and skeletal malformations and adverse effects on the male reproductive system in animal studies. This only occurred at doses greater than 190 (Asacol) and greater than 80 (Asacol HD) times the human dose based on body surface area. A Danish cohort study did not show any teratogenic effects of aminosalicylates in general during pregnancy.[27] Sulfasalazine readily crosses the placenta but has not been associated with any fetal abnormalities. Women taking sulfasalazine should be supplemented with folate daily. Topical 5-ASA products are also safe in pregnancy.[28]

Breastfeeding

Breastfeeding is low risk with exposure to sulfasalazine. The levels of transfer to breast milk are negligible. A rare association with diarrhea in the infant has been reported.[29] Therefore, the infant can be monitored for diarrhea if the mother is on aminosalicylates. Unlike other sulfonamides, there is no risk of kernicterus with aminosalicylates, as there is no displacement of

Table 7-1

Medication Recommendations for Pregnancy and Breast Feeding

	FDA Pregnancy Category*	Pregnancy Comment	Breastfeeding Comment
5-ASA			
Sulfasalazine	B	Low risk, replace folate daily	Probably compatible, possible diarrhea in infant
Mesalamine (Asacol, Asacol HD)	C	Low risk: possible skeletal and male reproductive abnormalities in animal studies, consider alternate 5-ASA	Probably compatible, DBP in coating is excreted into breast milk, unknown effects
Mesalamine (all other brands)	B	Low risk	Probably compatible, possible diarrhea in infant
Olsalazine	C	Low risk	Probably compatible, possible diarrhea in infant
Balsalazide	B	Low risk	Probably compatible, possible diarrhea in infant
Corticosteroids	C	Low risk: possible increased risk of cleft palate, adrenal insufficiency, premature rupture of membranes	Compatible
Antibiotics			
Metronidazole	B	Low risk, possibly avoid first trimester	Potential toxicity with higher doses and longer duration

(continued)

Table 7-1 *(continued)*

Medication Recommendations for Pregnancy and Breast Feeding

	FDA Pregnancy Category*	Pregnancy Comment	Breastfeeding Comment
Quinolones	C	Avoid, potential damage to cartilage	Probably compatible in short courses
Amoxicillin/ clavulanate	B	Low risk	Probably compatible
Cephalosporins	B	Low risk	Compatible
Immunomodulators			
6-MP/ Azathioprine	D	Low risk, animal teratogen	Probably compatible, consider discarding breast milk produced in the 4 hours after dosing
Methotrexate	X	Contraindicated, teratogenic to humans	Contraindicated, immunosuppression
Cyclosporine	C	Low risk	Potential toxicity, immunosuppression
Thalidomide	X	Contraindicated, teratogenic to humans	Contraindicated
Biologics			
Infliximab	B	Low risk, consider dosing close to 30 to 32 weeks and then after delivery	Probably compatible

(continued)

Table 7-1 *(continued)*

Medication Recommendations for Pregnancy and Breast Feeding

	FDA Pregnancy Category*	Pregnancy Comment	Breastfeeding Comment
Adalimumab	B	Low risk, consider dosing at week 32 and after delivery	Probably compatible
Certolizumab pegol	B	Low risk, continue dosing through pregnancy	Probably compatible
Natalizumab	C	Low risk	Probably compatible

Adapted from Kwan LY, Mahadevan U. Inflammatory bowel disease and pregnancy: an update. *Expert Review of Clinical Immunology.* 2010;6.4:643-657 and Mahadevan U, Kane S. American Gastroenterological Association Institute medical position statement on the use of gastrointestinal medications in pregnancy. *Gastroenterology.* 2006;131(1):278-282.
*See Appendix for discussion of FDA pregnancy categories.

bilirubin. Dibutyl phthalate, an inactive ingredient in the enteric coating of Asacol and Asacol HD tablets, and its primary metabolite monobutyl phthalate are also excreted into human milk. The clinical significance of the excretion of dibutyl phthalate and monobutyl phthalate into human milk has not been established.

ANTIBIOTICS DURING PREGNANCY

Metronidazole is a Category B drug and is low risk during pregnancy. Several trials have supported this, including 2 meta-analyses[30,31] and cohort studies.[32,33] One case control study did demonstrate a possible increased risk of cleft palate with use in the first trimester[34]; however, the study could not account for recall bias. The authors ultimately concluded that treatment with oral metronidazole during pregnancy presented no clinically important association with congenital abnormalities.[34] First trimester use was also not associated with birth defects in meta-analysis.[30] Therefore, therapy with metronidazole is considered safe during the course of pregnancy and should be used when indicated. Quinolones (eg, ciprofloxacin, levofloxacin, and norfloxacin) are Category C drugs. They are associated with potential damage to joints in children. In general, these medications should be avoided in pregnancy. However, studies in humans have not shown an increased risk of congenital malformations in children exposed during pregnancy.[35,36] A recent meta-analysis of quinolone use during the first trimester of pregnancy was also reassuring, with no increased risk of major malformation, stillbirth, preterm birth, or low birth weight.[37] Ampicillin, erythromycin, amoxicillin/clavulanic acid, and cephalosporins are antibiotics believed to be safe in pregnancy. Recent data from the National Birth Defects Prevention Study were reassuring, in that, while penicillins, erythromycins, and cephalosporins were commonly used during pregnancy, these medications were not associated with many birth defects.[38]

Breastfeeding

According to the American Academy of Pediatrics, metronidazole should be withheld for 12 to 24 hours if a single high dose of metronidazole is given because it is transferred in breast milk.[16] Long-term use while breastfeeding is not recommended. There are limited data on quinolones and breastfeeding, although they are likely safe to use if absolutely indicated. Amoxicillin/clavulanic acid is believed to be safe during breastfeeding.

CORTICOSTEROIDS DURING PREGNANCY

Corticosteroids are Category C drugs. A meta-analysis from 2000 showed a mild increased risk of cleft palate associated with first trimester use. There were no significant risks of major malformations.[39] A cohort study since this time of women with first trimester use of corticosteroids demonstrated no significant increased risk of major malformations and no cleft palate.[40] Therefore, when needed to control disease activity, corticosteroids can be used. The use of budesonide is not recommended over prednisone in pregnancy.

Breastfeeding

Limited data show that corticosteroids are probably safe to use during breastfeeding. There are no data on budesonide and breastfeeding.

AZATHIOPRINE/6-MERCAPTOPURINE (THIOPURINE CLASS) DURING PREGNANCY

Six-mercaptopurine (6-MP) and its prodrug azathioprine (AZA) are Category D drugs. Much of the early data on these drugs comes from animal studies and from the transplantation literature, which shows that 6-MP/AZA is teratogenic in animals and that rates of congenital anomalies ranged from 0% to 11.8% without recurrent patterns.[41] In one series of IBD patients, there was no increase in congenital anomalies associated with 6-MP/AZA use.[42,43] A recent large cohort study of pregnant women with IBD also demonstrated no increased risk of congenital anomalies associated with thiopurine use.[44] A long-term follow-up study of children exposed to azathioprine in utero or via breastfeeding with assessment at a median of 3.3 years showed no increase in infectious risk for children.[45] In general, it is thought that 6-MP/AZA can be used safely in pregnancy if necessary, particularly in the IBD population where the risks to mother and fetus due to flare of disease are known to be significant.

Breastfeeding

There is no absolute contraindication to breastfeeding while on AZA/6-MP, and 2 recent studies are reassuring. Sau and colleagues collected 31 breast milk samples from 10 women and measured 6-MP levels in the range of 0 to 18 hours postingestion. They found undetectable levels of 6-MP in all samples except 2 from one woman. These samples had levels of 1.2 and 7.6 µg/L and were taken at 3 and 6 hours, respectively, postthiopurine ingestion. In addition, 6-MP and 6-TGN were undetectable in neonatal blood.[46] Christensen and colleagues studied 8 lactating women on azathioprine and measured plasma and breast milk concentrations at hourly intervals for the first 5 hours after ingestion of the medication. The major part of 6-MP in breast milk was found within the first 4 hours after ingestion, at low levels overall (2 to 50 µg/L). Based on these findings, the authors concluded that breastfeeding is safe and that, to minimize the possibility of fetal exposure, consideration could be given to using a breast pump to discard the first portion of milk after thiopurine ingestion.[47] A recent study on the long-term follow-up of babies exposed in utero or via breastfeeding to azathioprine also did not show any increased risk of infection.[45] In general, breastfeeding during treatment with thiopurines is safe and should be recommended considering the known benefits of breast milk for the neonate.

CYCLOSPORINE DURING PREGNANCY

Cyclosporine is a Category C drug and overall is a low risk drug to use in pregnancy. In the setting of steroid-refractory fulminant UC, it can be considered as an alternative medical treatment to colectomy when surgical therapy may pose a risk to the mother and fetus. A meta-analysis showed no significant increase in congenital malformations associated with cyclosporine use. The overall rate of malformations was 4.1%, which is similar to the general population.[48]

Breastfeeding

According to the American Academy of Pediatrics, cyclosporine is contraindicated in breastfeeding due to potential for immunosuppression and neutropenia. It is excreted in breast milk in high concentrations.[49]

BIOLOGIC THERAPY

INFLIXIMAB DURING PREGNANCY

Infliximab is a pregnancy Category B drug and is used for induction and maintenance therapy in CD and UC. It is a chimeric anti-TNF monoclonal IgG_1 antibody that does not cross the placenta in the first trimester. It does cross the placenta in the second and third trimesters, and it is detectable in the infant several months after birth. It is not associated with an increased risk for congenital anomalies or infectious complications in children born to mothers receiving therapy.[50,51] However, levels in neonates can be detected up to 6 months of age. Therefore, it is recommended that live vaccines be avoided in the first 6 months (the only current recommended live vaccine in the first 6 months is the rotavirus vaccine). Infliximab should be continued during conception and the first and second trimester on schedule. Current convention for use of infliximab, if the patient is in remission, is that the last dose should be given around week 30 to 32 of gestation and then immediately after delivery (which may reduce transmission in the third trimester to the fetus).

Breastfeeding

Infliximab is safe to use during breastfeeding. In a study by Kane and colleagues, mothers with CD on infliximab were followed prospectively. No detectable levels of infliximab were found in breast milk in spite of detectable levels in mothers' serum.[52]

ADALIMUMAB DURING PREGNANCY

Adalimumab is a Category B drug approved for induction and maintenance of remission in CD. Adalimumab is an IgG_1 antibody and would be expected to cross the placenta in the third trimester as infliximab does. In a recent study, Mahadevan and colleagues showed transmission of adalimumab across the placenta, with detectable levels of drug in the cord blood of 5 infants whose mothers were taking adalimumab.[53] In all cases, the level in the infant's cord blood was higher than that in the mother. Interestingly, the level in the cord blood did not necessarily correlate with the date of cessation of adalimumab.[53] In a patient with CD in remission, the last dose of adalimumab can be given at week 32 of gestation and then immediately after delivery so as to minimize fetal levels at birth. However, given recent data indicating the lack of correlation with date of cessation and cord blood levels, one could also consider continuing adalimumab without cessation. As with infliximab, the infant should avoid live vaccines in the first 6 months of life due to the possibility of residual drug.

Breastfeeding

Adalimumab is considered safe in breastfeeding, although there are no trials in humans.

CERTOLIZUMAB PEGOL DURING PREGNANCY

Certolizumab pegol is a PEGylated Fab' fragment of a humanized anti-TNF-α monoclonal antibody that is used for induction and maintenance of remission in CD. A Category B drug, it does not have an Fc portion and therefore is not expected to be actively transported across the placenta as are infliximab and adalimumab. Given its minimal placental transfer, certolizumab can be continued on schedule until delivery. It may not be necessary to withhold live vaccines in the first 6 months from infants whose mothers were maintained on certolizumab pegol throughout pregnancy, as there is minimal transfer across the placenta.[54]

Breastfeeding

Certolizumab pegol is considered safe in breastfeeding, although there are no trials in humans.

NATALIZUMAB DURING PREGNANCY

Natalizumab is a recombinant humanized monoclonal IgG4 antibody against the α-unit of integrins (α4β1 and α4β7). These integrins are expressed on leukocytes, except for neutrophils. It blocks the adhesion and subsequent migration of the leukocytes into the target tissue by binding to α4-integrin. It is a Category C drug, and data on use in pregnancy are limited. A recent case report of 2 patients treated with natalizumab for multiple sclerosis by Hoeveneran and colleagues described delivery of healthy babies after natalizumab exposure.[55] No drug levels were available from serum or cord blood. Mahadevan and colleagues also published an abstract using data from the company on 143 pregnancies with natalizumab exposure.[56] No congenital malformations were reported. Of the 102 prospectively followed cases with known outcomes, there were 55 (53.4%) live births, 27 (26.2%) elective terminations, 21 (20.4%) spontaneous abortions, and no stillbirths.

Breastfeeding

Natalizumab transmission to breast milk is currently unknown. There are currently no trials in humans.

MANAGEMENT OF COMPLICATIONS

Ensuring remission prior to pregnancy is the best way to minimize potential complications associated with pregnancy. The presence of active disease is associated with continued or worsening disease activity in 70% of women.[57] Exacerbations of IBD should be managed aggressively to avoid serious complications, such as fulminant colitis, hemorrhage, perforation, premature labor, or fetal demise.

Diagnostic studies used to assess the patient with IBD include radiologic studies and endoscopic procedures, both of which must be carefully considered when dealing with the pregnant patient. If, however, it is necessary to perform these procedures, it should be recommended after discussion with the patient of the risks and benefits associated with the procedure.

LABORATORY STUDIES

As with all IBD patients on immunomodulator therapy and biologics, monitoring with routine lab studies should be continued. The normal physiologic changes of pregnancy should be considered when evaluating lab results. Inflammatory markers, such as erythrocyte sedimentation rate and C-reactive protein, may be elevated in pregnancy. Liver function tests, particularly the alkaline phosphatase, may also be elevated.[58] In addition, blood volume increases from 6 to 35 weeks gestation, resulting in a hemodilution of pregnancy. There may also be an increase in red cell mass, variable leukocyte counts, and a rise in platelet counts, but the rise should remain within normal limits.

RADIOLOGIC STUDIES

A variety of radiologic studies are available to evaluate for potential complications associated with IBD including bowel obstructions or abscesses. In choosing the appropriate radiology study, the clinician must not only consider which test would best identify the abnormality, but also must take into consideration whether the test emits ionizing radiation and how far along in the pregnancy the patient is in order to avoid risks to the fetus. Diagnostic studies that emit ionizing radiation include plain films, CT scans, and barium studies. A single radiologic procedure does not result in significant enough radiation exposure to harm the fetus[59]; however, the first trimester is the period in which radiation exposure can induce growth, mental retardation, and cancer.[60] MRI and ultrasound do not emit ionizing radiation and, therefore, are the radiologic studies of choice in the pregnant patient. However, gadolinium chelates have been shown to cross the placenta, and so the use of MRI with contrast in the first trimester is not recommended. Nonemergent radiologic procedures should be avoided if possible during pregnancy, particularly during the first trimester, but, if necessary, they can be performed safely.

KEY POINTS

- Nonemergent radiologic procedures should be avoided if possible.
- Initial tests can include ultrasound and MRI, which do not emit ionizing radiation.
- If other radiologic tests are needed, avoid first trimester exposure if possible.
- A single radiologic procedure does not result in enough radiation exposure to harm the fetus.

ENDOSCOPIC PROCEDURES

Endoscopy is a valuable tool to assess the anatomic extent of IBD. Flexible sigmoidoscopy is thought to be a safe procedure during pregnancy, when performed in the second trimester (see Chapter 8). In a study of 24 pregnant patients who underwent 26 sigmoidoscopies, there were no complications associated with the actual procedure. All reported poor fetal outcomes were in high-risk pregnancies and were not temporally related to the procedure. This suggests that, in clinically stable pregnancies, sigmoidoscopy is a safe procedure.[61] Similar results have been observed in other studies. Esophagogastroduodenoscopy (EGD) is occasionally necessary as well in the evaluation of the IBD patient and is also thought to be a safe procedure.[62] Colonoscopy should be avoided in pregnancy except when strongly indicated. A recent study by Cappell and colleagues on colonoscopy during pregnancy found that the procedure may be relatively safe and without large fetal risks when performed during the second trimester.[63] Excessive sedation should be minimized, and procedures should be performed by an experienced endoscopist when these procedures are needed.

KEY POINTS

- Flexible sigmoidoscopy can be safely performed in the second trimester, if needed.
- Colonoscopy should be avoided unless strongly indicated; recent data have shown relative safety of colonoscopy in the second trimester.
- Excessive sedation should be avoided.
- Procedures should be performed by an experienced endoscopist.

SURGERY

Treating IBD with medications is the optimal way of managing the pregnant IBD patient. However, life-threatening complications such as toxic megacolon, fulminant colitis, or intestinal obstruction may rarely require surgical intervention. The health and safety of both mother and fetus must be considered when deciding the optimal time to perform surgery. The second trimester has been shown to be safe for women in the general population to undergo routine nonobstetrical surgical procedures, and surgeries have also been performed in the third trimester without preterm delivery.

For UC patients with fulminant colitis, options for management include Turnbull-Blowhole colostomy and subtotal colectomy. Turnbull-Blowhole colostomy, used for colonic decompression with the formation of a loop ileostomy, is a relatively safe surgical procedure.[64] Patients undergo restorative proctocolectomy and IPAA at a later date. Case reports have shown that third-trimester colectomies for severe colitis have been successful when surgery has been combined with C-section or with later vaginal delivery.[65-67] Haq and colleagues suggest that patients less than 28 weeks gestation undergo a Turnbull-Blowhole colostomy and those greater than 28 weeks undergo a synchronous C-section and subtotal colectomy, if possible.[68]

The indications for surgery in CD include intestinal obstruction or perforation, hemorrhage, or abscess. Temporary ileostomy is preferred to reduce the risk of postoperative complications that can be seen after primary anastomosis. Surgery should not be avoided or prolonged due to the patient being pregnant, as concerns for fetal loss appear to be related to the severity of the maternal disease and not the surgery itself.[69]

KEY POINTS
• Medical therapy rather than surgery is optimal during pregnancy.
• Health and safety of both mother and fetus need to be considered when determining timing of surgery.
• For UC patients with fulminant colitis, options include Turnbull-Blowhole colostomy and subtotal colectomy.
• Indications for surgery in CD include obstruction, perforation, hemorrhage, or abscess.
• Temporary ileostomy is preferred surgery in CD to reduce complication risks of primary anastomosis.

NUTRITION IN THE PREGNANT INFLAMMATORY BOWEL DISEASE PATIENT

Clinically diagnosed protein-calorie malnutrition is rare in the non-IBD pregnant patient; however, a study by Nguyen and colleagues[4] found a 20-fold higher likelihood of malnutrition among women with CD and a 60-fold likelihood of malnutrition among women with UC. A study by Moser and colleagues has also shown that women with CD gained less weight during pregnancy than non-IBD patients.[16] These findings highlight the need for nutritional screening to detect signs of undernutrition or malnutrition in pregnant IBD patients to avoid perinatal morbidity and mortality.

Several factors contribute to the development and progression of malnutrition in patients with IBD. In patients with UC, there may be more of a precipitous course with a rapid growth of acute nutritional development after an initial presentation of relatively good nutritional status. In CD, malnutrition may develop slowly over time, and patients often have multiple, severe nutritional deficiencies. Several factors can contribute to malnutrition in IBD patients. Decreased nutrient intake from anorexia and malabsorption and nutrient losses resulting from intestinal inflammation or ulceration have been implicated as causes of malnutrition. Extensive inflammation or ulceration can limit small intestinal absorptive surface area. In addition, increased protein and energy requirements from a catabolic state[70] as well as some of the medications used in the treatment of IBD such as sulfasalazine and corticosteroids can also contribute to the development of nutrient deficiencies.

Common vitamin and mineral deficiencies in IBD patients include folate, vitamin A, vitamin D, vitamin B_{12}, iron, magnesium, and zinc. Folic acid supplementation is recommended for all pregnant patients; however, IBD patients may be taking medications such as sulfasalazine that interfere with folic acid metabolism. Pregnant IBD patients should take folic acid supplements of at least 2 mg/day instead of the 1 mg/day recommended for the non-IBD patient. Patients requiring corticosteroid treatment should be supplemented with vitamin D and calcium to avoid vitamin D deficiency and to decrease the risk of osteoporosis. Many patients with CD have inflammation affecting the small bowel or have undergone ileal resections, which may cause bile salt and vitamin B_{12} malabsorption, leading to bile salt depletion and consequent fat and fat-soluble vitamin malabsorption. Vitamin B_{12} supplementation should be considered.

If necessary, both enteral nutrition and total parenteral nutrition can and have been used to support the pregnant IBD patient.[16,20,71] Parenteral nutrition is indicated to correct severe nutrition when there are contraindications to enteral nutrition or when enteral nutrition is unsuccessful. Elemental diets have also been safely used in pregnancy, both as a primary therapy for active CD and as a source for supplemental nutrition.[72]

KEY POINTS

- Common deficiencies include folate, vitamin A, vitamin D, vitamin B_{12}, iron, magnesium, and zinc.
- Folate supplementation in the pregnant patient on sulfasalazine should be 2 mg/day.
- Enteral nutrition and parenteral nutrition can be used when necessary.

MODE OF DELIVERY

Prior studies have demonstrated an increased risk of C-section among women with IBD. In the 1990s, Kornfeld reported a C-section rate of 15% for women with IBD as compared to 10% among the non-IBD population.[17] In a recent cohort from the Netherlands, the rate of C-section among women with IBD was 32%. Women with perianal disease had increased odds of caesarean delivery (OR: 4.6; 95% CI: 1.8 to 11.4).[15] Another recent United States study confirmed this increased risk of C-section in both women with CD and UC (CD OR: 1.72; 95% CI: 1.44 to 2.04 and UC OR: 1.29; 95% CI: 1.01 to 1.66).[4] Current recommendations are for delivery by C-section for those women with active perianal disease at the time of delivery and to consider C-section in those patients with IPAA. Vaginal delivery has been shown to exacerbate perianal disease in patients with active disease at the time of delivery. This is likely related to perianal or anal sphincter damage.[73] In women with IPAA prior to pregnancy, C-section is recommended if the perineum is scarred, causing it to be rigid and less compliant. This decreases the risk of incontinence and damage to anal sphincters. Pouch dysfunction with vaginal delivery is a concern; however, there are data to suggest that vaginal delivery is low risk for those with a pouch, as there is generally a return to prepregnancy function within 6 months.[74] In the absence of perianal disease or IPAA, mode of delivery is at the discretion of the obstetrician.

KEY POINTS
• C-section is more common among women with IBD. • Indications for C-section include active perianal disease and prior IPAA. • Mode of delivery for patients with IBD should be at the discretion of the obstetrician.

SUMMARY

The peak incidence of IBD in women occurs during the reproductive years. Because of this, the influences of IBD on pregnancy and pregnancy on IBD become very important. Comanagement of the pregnant IBD patient by both a gastroenterologist and an obstetrician is necessary. The goals of management of the pregnant IBD patient are similar to those of the nonpregnant patient: to induce and maintain remission. The health of the mother is the most important factor for the health of the baby. Because of this, the risk-benefit ratio of continuing medications for IBD most often supports the continuation of IBD-specific medications during pregnancy. Nutrition is important in patients with IBD and becomes more so in the pregnant patient. Optimizing nutritional status benefits both the mother and the fetus. The need for endoscopic testing and/or surgery during pregnancy is individually decided based on the clinical scenario. In general, the second trimester is the optimal time for these procedures if they are absolutely indicated. Decisions for mode of delivery should be determined for obstetric reasons except in those with active perianal disease or with a history of IPAA, where C-section is often indicated to prevent damage to the anal sphincter. Decisions for continuation of IBD-specific medications during breastfeeding are made on an individual basis, although many of the medications used for IBD are considered safe with lactation. In general, outcomes of pregnancies in IBD patients are similar to those of the general population, with a somewhat increased risk of being small for gestational age and preterm labor, particularly among those with active disease during pregnancy.

REFERENCES

1. Andres PG, Friedman LS. Epidemiology and the natural course of inflammatory bowel disease. *Gastroenterol Clin North Am.* 1999;28(2):255-281, vii.
2. Baiocco PJ, Korelitz BI. The influence of inflammatory bowel disease and its treatment on pregnancy and fetal outcome. *J Clin Gastroenterol.* 1984;6(3): 211-216.
3. Raatikainen K, Mustonen J, Pajala MO, Heikkinen M, Heinonen S. The effects of pre- and post-pregnancy inflammatory bowel disease diagnosis on birth outcomes. *Aliment Pharmacol Ther.* 2011;33(3):333-339.
4. Nguyen GC, Boudreau H, Harris ML, Maxwell CV. Outcomes of obstetric hospitalizations among women with inflammatory bowel disease in the United States. *Clin Gastroenterol Hepatol.* 2009;7(3):329-334.
5. Kwan LY, Mahadevan U. Inflammatory bowel disease and pregnancy: an update. *Expert Rev Clin Immunol.* 2010;6(4):643-657.
6. Mountifield R, Bampton P, Prosser R, Muller K, Andrews JM. Fear and fertility in inflammatory bowel disease: a mismatch of perception and reality affects family planning decisions. *Inflamm Bowel Dis.* 2009;15(5):720-725.

7. Willoughby CP, Truelove SC. UC and pregnancy. *Gut.* 1980;21(6):469-474.

8. Olsen KO, Joelsson M, Laurberg S, Oresland T. Fertility after ileal pouch-anal anastomosis in women with UC. *Br J Surg.* 1999;86(4):493-495.

9. Waljee A, Waljee J, Morris AM, Higgins PD. Threefold increased risk of infertility: a meta-analysis of infertility after ileal pouch anal anastomosis in UC. *Gut.* 2006;55(11):1575-1580.

10. Orholm M, Fonager K, Sorensen HT. Risk of UC and Crohn's disease among offspring of patients with chronic inflammatory bowel disease. *Am J Gastroenterol.* 1999;94(11):3236-3238.

11. Moody GA, Mayberry JF. Perceived sexual dysfunction amongst patients with inflammatory bowel disease. *Digestion.* 1993;54(4):256-260.

12. Bennett RA, Rubin PH, Present DH. Frequency of inflammatory bowel disease in offspring of couples both presenting with inflammatory bowel disease. *Gastroenterology.* 1991;100(6):1638-1643.

13. Morales M, Berney T, Jenny A, Morel P, Extermann P. Crohn's disease as a risk factor for the outcome of pregnancy. *Hepatogastroenterology.* 2000;47(36):1595-1598.

14. Nielsen OH, Andreasson B, Bondesen S, Jacobsen O, Jarnum S. Pregnancy in Crohn's disease. *Scand J Gastroenterol.* 1984;19(6):724-732.

15. Smink M, Lotgering FK, Albers L, de Jong DJ. Effect of childbirth on the course of Crohn's disease; results from a retrospective cohort study in the Netherlands. *BMC Gastroenterol.* 2011;11:6.

16. Moser MA, Okun NB, Mayes DC, Bailey RJ. Crohn's disease, pregnancy, and birth weight. *Am J Gastroenterol.* 2000;95(4):1021-1026.

17. Kornfeld D, Cnattingius S, Ekbom A. Pregnancy outcomes in women with inflammatory bowel disease—a population-based cohort study. *Am J Obstet Gynecol.* 1997;177(4):942-946.

18. Mahadevan U, Sandborn WJ, Li DK, Hakimian S, Kane S, Corley DA. Pregnancy outcomes in women with inflammatory bowel disease: a large community-based study from Northern California. *Gastroenterology.* 2007; 133(4):1106-1112.

19. Cornish J, Tan E, Teare J, et al. A meta-analysis on the influence of inflammatory bowel disease on pregnancy. *Gut.* 2007;56(6):830-837.

20. Nielsen OH, Andreasson B, Bondesen S, Jarnum S. Pregnancy in ulcerative colitis. *Scand J Gastroenterol.* 1983;18(6):735-742.

21. Nelson JL, Hughes KA, Smith AG, Nisperos BB, Branchaud AM, Hansen JA. Maternal-fetal disparity in HLA class II alloantigens and the pregnancy-induced amelioration of rheumatoid arthritis. *N Engl J Med.* 1993;329(7):466-471.

22. Agret F, Cosnes J, Hassani Z, et al. Impact of pregnancy on the clinical activity of Crohn's disease. *Aliment Pharmacol Ther.* 2005;21(5):509-513.

23. Castiglione F, Pignata S, Morace F, et al. Effect of pregnancy on the clinical course of a cohort of women with inflammatory bowel disease. *Ital J Gastroenterol.* 1996;28(4):199-204.

24. Kane S, Lemieux N. The role of breastfeeding in postpartum disease activity in women with inflammatory bowel disease. *Am J Gastroenterol.* 2005;100(1):102-105.

25. Moffatt DC, Ilnyckyj A, Bernstein CN. A population-based study of breastfeeding in inflammatory bowel disease: initiation, duration, and effect on disease in the postpartum period. *Am J Gastroenterol.* 2009;104(10):2517-2523.

26. Mahadevan U, Kane S. American Gastroenterological Association Institute medical position statement on the use of gastrointestinal medications in pregnancy. *Gastroenterology.* 2006;131(1):278-282.

27. Norgard B, Fonager K, Pedersen L, Jacobsen BA, Sorensen HT. Birth outcome in women exposed to 5-aminosalicylic acid during pregnancy: a Danish cohort study. *Gut.* 2003;52(2):243-247.

28. Habal FM, Hui G, Greenberg GR. Oral 5-aminosalicylic acid for inflammatory bowel disease in pregnancy: safety and clinical course. *Gastroenterology.* 1993;105(4):1057-1060.

29. Nelis GF. Diarrhoea due to 5-aminosalicylic acid in breast milk. *Lancet.* 1989;1:383.

30. Burtin P, Taddio A, Ariburnu O, Einarson TR, Koren G. Safety of metronidazole in pregnancy: a meta-analysis. *Am J Obstet Gynecol.* 1995;172(2, pt 1):525-529.

31. Caro-Paton T, Carvajal A, Martin de Diego I, Martin-Arias LH, Alvarez Requejo A, Rodriguez Pinilla E. Is metronidazole teratogenic? A meta-analysis. *Br J Clin Pharmacol.* 1997;44(2):179-182.

32. Piper JM, Mitchel EF, Ray WA. Prenatal use of metronidazole and birth defects: no association. *Obstet Gynecol.* 1993;82(3):348-352.

33. Sorensen HT, Larsen H, Jensen ES, et al. Safety of metronidazole during pregnancy: a cohort study of risk of congenital abnormalities, preterm delivery and low birth weight in 124 women. *J Antimicrob Chemother.* 1999;44(6):854-856.

34. Czeizel AE, Rockenbauer M. A population based case-control teratologic study of oral metronidazole treatment during pregnancy. *Br J Obstet Gynaecol.* 1998;105(3):322-327.

35. Larsen H, Nielsen GL, Schonheyder HC, Olesen C, Sorensen HT. Birth outcome following maternal use of fluoroquinolones. *Int J Antimicrob Agents.* 2001;18(3):259-262.

36. Loebstein R, Addis A, Ho E, et al. Pregnancy outcome following gestational exposure to fluoroquinolones: a multicenter prospective controlled study. *Antimicrob Agents Chemother.* 1998;42(6):1336-1339.

37. Bar-Oz B, Moretti ME, Boskovic R, O'Brien L, Koren G. The safety of quinolones—a meta-analysis of pregnancy outcomes. *Eur J Obstet Gynecol Reprod Biol.* 2009;143(2):75-78.

38. Crider KS, Cleves MA, Reefhuis J, Berry RJ, Hobbs CA, Hu DJ. Antibacterial medication use during pregnancy and risk of birth defects: National Birth Defects Prevention Study. *Arch Pediatr Adolesc Med.* 2009;163(11):978-985.

39. Park-Wyllie L, Mazzotta P, Pastuszak A, et al. Birth defects after maternal exposure to corticosteroids: prospective cohort study and meta-analysis of epidemiological studies. *Teratology.* 2000;62(6):385-392.

40. Hviid A, Molgaard-Nielsen D. Corticosteroid use during pregnancy and risk of orofacial clefts. *CMAJ.* 2011;183(7):796-804.

41. Polifka JE, Friedman JM. Teratogen update: azathioprine and 6-mercaptopurine. *Teratology.* 2002;65(5):240-261.

42. Francella A, Dyan A, Bodian C, Rubin P, Chapman M, Present DH. The safety of 6-mercaptopurine for childbearing patients with inflammatory bowel disease: a retrospective cohort study. *Gastroenterology.* 2003;124(1):9-17.

43. Moskovitz DN, Bodian C, Chapman ML, et al. The effect on the fetus of medications used to treat pregnant inflammatory bowel-disease patients. *Am J Gastroenterol.* 2004;99(4):656-661.
44. Coelho J, Beaugerie L, Colombel JF, et al. Pregnancy outcome in patients with inflammatory bowel disease treated with thiopurines: cohort from the CESAME Study. *Gut.* 2011;60(2):198-203.
45. Angelberger S, Reinisch W, Messerschmidt A, et al. Long-term follow-up of babies exposed to azathioprine in utero and via breastfeeding. *J Crohns Colitis.* 2011;5(2):95-100.
46. Sau A, Clarke S, Bass J, Kaiser A, Marinaki A, Nelson-Piercy C. Azathioprine and breastfeeding: is it safe? *BJOG.* 2007;114(4):498-501.
47. Christensen LA, Dahlerup JF, Nielsen MJ, Fallingborg JF, Schmiegelow K. Azathioprine treatment during lactation. *Aliment Pharmacol Ther.* 2008;28(10):1209-1213.
48. Bar Oz B, Hackman R, Einarson T, Koren G. Pregnancy outcome after cyclosporine therapy during pregnancy: a meta-analysis. *Transplantation.* 2001;71(8):1051-1055.
49. American Academy of Pediatrics Committee on Drugs. Transfer of drugs and other chemicals into human milk. *Pediatrics.* 2001; 108(3):776-789.
50. Katz JA, Antoni C, Keenan GF, Smith DE, Jacobs SJ, Lichtenstein GR. Outcome of pregnancy in women receiving infliximab for the treatment of Crohn's disease and rheumatoid arthritis. *Am J Gastroenterol.* 2004;99(12):2385-2392.
51. Mahadevan U, Kane S, Sandborn WJ, et al. Intentional infliximab use during pregnancy for induction or maintenance of remission in Crohn's disease. *Aliment Pharmacol Ther.* 2005;21(6):733-738.
52. Kane S, Ford J, Cohen R, Wagner C. Absence of infliximab in infants and breast milk from nursing mothers receiving therapy for Crohn's disease before and after delivery. *J Clin Gastroenterol.* 2009;43(7):613-616.
53. Mahadevan U, Miller JK, Wolf DC. Adalimumab levels detected in cord blood and infants exposed in utero. *Gastroenterology.* 2011;140:S61-S62.
54. Mahadevan U, Abreu MT. Certolizumab use in pregnancy: Low levels detected in cord blood. *Gastroenterology.* 2009;136(5 suppl 1):A146-A147.
55. Hoevenaren IA, de Vries LC, Rijnders RJP, Lotgering FK. Delivery of healthy babies after natalizumab use for multiple sclerosis: a report of two cases. Acta Neurol Scand: 2011: 123(6): 430–433.
56. Mahadevan U, Nazareth M, Cristiano L, et al. Natalizumab use during pregnancy. Am J Gastroenterol. 2008;103:P295.
57. *Pregnancy in Gastrointestinal Disorders.* Bethesda, MD: American College of Gastroenterology. URL: http://s3.gi.org/physicians/PregnancyMonograph.pdf.
58. Abbassi-Ghanavati M, Greer LG, Cunningham FG. Pregnancy and laboratory studies: a reference table for clinicians. *Obstet Gynecol.* 2009;114(6):1326-1331.
59. Hall EJ. Scientific view of low-level radiation risks. *Radiographics.* 1991;11(3):509-518.
60. Nicklas AH, Baker ME. Imaging strategies in the pregnant cancer patient. *Semin Oncol.* 2000;27(6):623-632.

61. Cappell MS, Colon VJ, Sidhom OA. A study at 10 medical centers of the safety and efficacy of 48 flexible sigmoidoscopies and 8 colonoscopies during pregnancy with follow-up of fetal outcome and with comparison to control groups. *Dig Dis Sci.* 1996;41(12):2353-2361.

62. Cappell MS. The fetal safety and clinical efficacy of gastrointestinal endoscopy during pregnancy. *Gastroenterol Clin North Am.* 2003;32(1):123-179.

63. Cappell MS, Fox SR, Gorrepati N. Safety and efficacy of colonoscopy during pregnancy: an analysis of pregnancy outcome in 20 patients. *J Reprod Med.* 2010;55(3-4):115-123.

64. Ooi BS, Remzi FH, Fazio VW. Turnbull-Blowhole colostomy for toxic UC in pregnancy: report of two cases. *Dis Colon Rectum.* 2003; 46(1):111-115.

65. Watson WJ, Gaines TE. Third-trimester colectomy for severe UC. A case report. *J Reprod Med.* 1987;32(11):869-872.

66. Bohe MG, Ekelund GR, Genell SN, et al. Surgery for fulminating colitis during pregnancy. *Dis Colon Rectum.* 1983;26(2):119-122.

67. Boulton R, Hamilton M, Lewis A, Walker P, Pounder R. Fulminant UC in pregnancy. *Am J Gastroenterol.* 1994;89(6):931-933.

68. Haq AI, Sahai A, Hallworth S, Rampton DS, Dorudi S. Synchronous colectomy and caesarean section for fulminant UC: case report and review of the literature. *Int J Colorectal Dis.* 2006;21(5):465-469.

69. Dubinsky M, Abraham B, Mahadevan U. Management of the pregnant IBD patient. *Inflamm Bowel Dis.* 2008;14(12):1736-1750.

70. Han PD, Burke A, Baldassano RN, Rombeau JL, Lichtenstein GR. Nutrition and inflammatory bowel disease. *Gastroenterol Clin North Am.* 1999;28(2):423-443, ix.

71. Miller JP. Inflammatory bowel disease in pregnancy: a review. *J R Soc Med.* 1986;79(4):221-225.

72. Teahon K, Pearson M, Levi AJ, Bjarnason I. Elemental diet in the management of Crohn's disease during pregnancy. *Gut.* 1991;32(9):1079-1081.

73. Ilnyckyji A, Blanchard JF, Rawsthorne P, Bernstein CN. Perianal Crohn's disease and pregnancy: role of the mode of delivery. *Am J Gastroenterol.* 1999;94(11):3274-3278.

74. Beniada A, Benoist G, Maurel J, Dreyfus M. [Inflammatory bowel disease and pregnancy: report of 76 cases and review of the literature]. *J Gynecol Obstet Biol Reprod (Paris).* 2005;34(6):581-588.

8

Endoscopy

Kim L. Isaacs, MD, PhD

Gastrointestinal endoscopy is an important diagnostic and thera-peutic tool in a large number of conditions involving the gastroin-testinal tract. These procedures including upper endoscopy, colonos-copy, and endoscopic retrograde cholangiopancreatography (ERCP) are relatively safe and well-tolerated in the general population. In the pregnant patient, there are risks that are related to both mother and fetus. The relative risks and benefits of these procedures in this patient population have not been studied to the same extent as in the nonpregnant population.[1] If the benefit outweighs the risk to the fetus, then endoscopy should be performed. It is estimated that annually in the United States there are more than 12,000 pregnant patients with a strong indication for esophagogastroduodenoscopy (EGD), more than 6000 for colonoscopy or sigmoidoscopy, and more than 1000 for ERCP.[2]

GENERAL CONSIDERATIONS

The American Society for Gastrointestinal Endoscopy (ASGE) has published guidelines to guide the use of endoscopy in the

Isaacs KL, Long MD.
*GI and Liver Disease During Pregnancy:
A Practical Approach (pp. 117-132).*
© 2013 Taylor & Francis Group

Table 8-1

The American Society for Gastrointestinal Endoscopy Guidelines for Endoscopy in the Pregnant Patient

1. Have strong indications for endoscopy, especially in the high-risk patient.

2. Second trimester is the optimal time for endoscopy. If possible, defer the procedure to this time period.

3. Use the lowest dose of medication needed to perform the procedure.

4. Use Category A or B drugs (realistically Category B because there are no A drugs) for sedation.

5. Use the shortest procedure time possible.

6. Avoid placing the patient on her back for the procedure. The left lateral decubitus position is safe for the procedure.

7. In patients who are at the stage in pregnancy where fetal heart sounds can be detected, assess pre- and postprocedure. In certain cases, monitor during the procedure.

8. Have obstetric support available, especially in the second and third trimesters.

9. Do not endoscope in patients with imminent delivery and obstetrical complications, such as placenta previa.

pregnant patient (Table 8-1).[3] The approach to the pregnant patient is first to make sure that there is a strong indication for endoscopic evaluation/therapy and then to carry out endoscopy as safely as possible for the mother and the fetus. The risks that must be considered include teratogenicity of the drugs used during endoscopy (including preps used for colonoscopy and sigmoidoscopy), medication-induced hypoxia and hypotension, induction of premature labor, and fetal trauma.

INDICATIONS

In pregnancy, the decision to proceed with an endoscopic procedure should be well-documented with consideration of the indication for the procedure (Table 8-2).

Table 8-2

Indications for Endoscopic Procedures During Pregnancy

EGD
- GI bleeding
- Intractable nausea and vomiting
- Severe midepigastric/upper abdominal pain

Sigmoidoscopy/Colonoscopy
- Lower GI bleeding with strong suspicion of colon mass
- Severe diarrhea with negative noninvasive evaluation
- Severe exacerbation of inflammatory bowel disease

ERCP
- Gallstone pancreatitis
- Documented cholelithiasis
- Biliary or pancreatic ductal injury

PEG
- Severe hyperemesis gravidarum
- Prolonged coma

KEY POINTS
• Endoscopy is safe during pregnancy if indicated.
• Document indications.
• Discuss risks and benefits with the patient.

TIMING

During pregnancy, there are distinct stages of development that the fetus goes through. Most organ development takes place in the first trimester. During the third week of gestation, the brain, spinal cord, and heart begin to develop, and the GI tract starts to form. During weeks 4 and 5, there is limb development and further brain development. Eyes and ears begin to form, and the heart now beats at a regular interval. By week 7 of gestation, all the major organs have begun to form. In this trimester of pregnancy, the main medication and endoscopic concerns are those of teratogenesis. During the second trimester, there is further maturing of the organs so that, by week 25 of gestation, the respiratory system has developed enough so gas exchange is possible. There is slow progressive uterine growth with the growth of the fetus. By the third trimester, there is continued development with rapid growth of the gravid uterus. In terms of the safety of endoscopy, if it is elective, the optimal time to sedate and perform an endoscopic procedure is in the second trimester. This avoids the period of organogenesis and avoids the later months where there may be more concern about trauma to the enlarging uterus and stimulation of preterm labor. In many cases, the endoscopic procedure is more urgent and, if strongly indicated, should be carried out regardless of the stage of pregnancy.

KEY POINT
• Try to do endoscopic procedures in the second trimester or postpartum when possible.

PREGNANCY CONSIDERATIONS

In general, procedures in pregnant patients are carried out similarly to the same procedure in nonpregnant patients. Preprocedural consultation with the patient's obstetrician is recommended to identify any particular concerns for the patient at her stage of pregnancy.

MONITORING

Standard monitoring should include assessment of blood pressure, cardiac rate/rhythm, and measurement of oxygen saturation. Fetal monitoring should be considered on a case-by-case basis. If the fetus is previable, then it is recommended that fetal heart tones be assessed at the beginning and the end of the procedure.[4] If the fetus is viable, consideration can be made of continuous fetal monitoring along with monitoring for uterine contractions.[4] This decision should be made in consultation with the obstetrician based on the degree of illness of the patient, the anticipated intervention, and the obstetrical course.

RESPIRATORY

The growing fetus is sensitive to maternal hypoxia and hypotension. Physiologically, during pregnancy there is a 20% increase in oxygen consumption and a 20% decrease in the mother's pulmonary functional reserve capacity (FRC). This may lead to a rapid decrease in maternal oxygen saturation during periods of hypoventilation or apnea.[5] Oxygen supplementation should be used during the procedure.

POSITIONING

In the second and third trimesters, the patient should not lie in the supine position during any component of the procedure, including both preparation and recovery. The enlarging gravid uterus can compress the aorta and the vena cava if the patient is in the supine position. This may cause decreased blood flow to the placenta. Typically, the patient is placed in the left lateral decubitus position. Alternatives include sitting up or placing a wedge under the right hip to create a "pelvic tilt."[3]

BOWEL PREPARATION

For colonoscopy and flexible sigmoidoscopy, some bowel cleansing will likely be necessary for adequate visualization of the colonic mucosa. Polyethylene glycol-electrolyte (PEG) solutions (GoLYTELY, MiraLAX) have not been studied in pregnancy and are considered Category C drugs for pregnancy.[3] Sodium phosphate preparations are also classified as Category C agents but lead to more fluid and electrolyte abnormalities and should not be used. For a limited distal evaluation of the colon, tap water enemas may be used for cleansing and are considered safe. Care must be taken to maintain hydration status during the colonoscopy prep due to the adverse effects of hypotension on the fetus by decreasing placental blood flow. In patients with a tenuous hydration status, IV fluids should be given during the preparation process.

KEY POINTS
• Avoid maternal hypoxia and hypotension; monitor blood pressure, cardiac rate and rhythm, and oxygen saturation. • Use oxygen supplementation during all procedures. • Avoid positioning the patient in a supine position. • Fetal and uterine monitoring should be done on a case-by-case basis. • PEG for colonic prep, if needed.

MEDICATIONS

SEDATIVES AND ANALGESICS

Sedation for endoscopy in the pregnant patient is targeted at reducing anxiety. If heavy levels of sedation are necessary for more complicated procedures, management by an anesthesiologist may be required. In general, Category B and C drugs are used for sedation. Category D drugs are used if the risk is clearly outweighed by the benefit. The safety of medications used in endoscopy during pregnancy and breastfeeding is shown in Table 8-3.

MEPERIDINE

Meperidine, a Category B drug, is a narcotic analgesic that is rapidly transferred across the placenta. Several large studies have shown no teratogenicity in the first trimester.[1] It is broken down to normeperidine, which has a long half-life and can accumulate with toxic effects to the patient if given repeatedly. With a low, nonrepetitive dose used for gastroenterology procedures, this is not likely to happen. It crosses the blood-brain barrier of the fetus more slowly than with morphine. If given at delivery, meperidine may depress neonatal respiration for several hours.[1] It can also diminish fetal heart beat variability for one hour after maternal administration. Due to the respiratory effects on the fetus, meperidine should not be used at high doses at term. The therapeutic goal should be

Table 8-3

Common Medications Used During Endoscopy

Medication	FDA Pregnancy Category*	Pregnancy Comment	Breastfeeding Comment
Sedatives			
Meperidine	B	Crosses the blood-brain barrier of the fetus more slowly than MSO4 Do not use repetitive high doses Do not use high doses at term	May be detected up to 24 hours after administration Use alternative
Morphine	C	No congenital abnormalities when used in first trimester Risk in third trimester or in high doses at term	Does cross into breast milk—no immediate adverse effects on newborn AAP considers compatible
Fentanyl	C	Rapid first pass clearance Avoid high doses Less respiratory depression of infant at term than with meperidine	At 10 hours, undetectable in breast milk Low oral bioavailability Compatible
Propofol	B	Potentially deeper levels of sedation—careful attention to avoiding maternal hypoxia	Excreted in breast milk with maximum concentration 4 to 5 hours after administration

(continued)

Table 8-3 *(continued)*

Common Medications Used During Endoscopy

Medication	FDA Pregnancy Category*	Pregnancy Comment	Breastfeeding Comment
Diazepam	D	Concentrated in fetal circulation Cleft palate in rats Avoid	Withhold nursing for 4 hours after administration
Midazolam	D	Does not concentrate in fetal circulation Safer than diazepam Avoid hypoxia in mother	Withhold nursing for 4 hours after first administration Consider pump and dump of first milk after procedure
Sedation Antagonists			
Naloxone	B	Crosses placenta rapidly Do not give to narcotic addicts	No data available
Flumazenil	C	Likely crosses the placenta but a very short half-life Maternal benefit when needed is felt to outweigh embryo/fetal risk	Probably compatible
Adjunctive Agents			
Topical lidocaine	B	IV crosses placenta quickly The effects of topical administration are less clear but likely limited exposure to fetus	Compatible—do not swallow

(continued)

Table 8-3 *(continued)*

Common Medications Used During Endoscopy

Medication	FDA Pregnancy Category*	Pregnancy Comment	Breastfeeding Comment
Simethicone	C	Few studies; probably safe	Compatible
Glucagon	B	Very low risk— does not cross placenta	Compatible
PEG	C	Avoid dehydration	Probably compatible
Antibiotics			
Cephalosporins Cefazolin	B	Single dose early in pregnancy limited to body fluids	Excreted into breast milk in very low concentrations Compatible
Ampicillin/ sulbactam	B	No embryotoxicity or teratogenicity in animal studies	Excreted into breast milk For a single dose for procedure, no need to wait for term infant, but might wait 6 to 8 hours if preterm
Ciprofloxacin	C	Human data suggest low risk Some suggest caution in first trimester	Excreted into milk Limited data, potential toxicity AAP compatible

*See Appendix for discussion of FDA pregnancy categories.

relaxation and analgesia without somnolence. Dosages used should be in the range of 50 to 75 mg. Meperidine is excreted into breast milk with detectable levels up to 24 hours after administration. No adverse effects have been described in these infants; however, alternative narcotics should be considered in the breastfeeding mother.[6]

FENTANYL

Fentanyl, a Category C drug, has a more rapid half-life than meperidine, and there is a high first pass clearance. There have been no teratogenic effects reported with fentanyl, although rat studies have shown impaired fertility and embryotoxicity at high doses given over multiple days. It is transferred through the placenta in the first and second trimesters.[6] There are fewer reports of fetal heart rate variability with fentanyl, and, if given close to delivery, there is less respiratory depression. One case of respiratory muscle rigidity related to fentanyl has been described in a newborn.[7] Fentanyl is excreted into the milk with the peak levels at 0.75 hours. At 10 hours, the levels are virtually undetectable.[8] There is low oral bioavailability, and fentanyl is considered compatible with breastfeeding by the American Academy of Pediatrics (AAP).

MORPHINE

There are no described teratogenic effects for the use of morphine (Category C) in the first trimester. Placental transfer is rapid, and chronic use may lead to newborn addiction. Use in limited amounts in endoscopy is likely safe. If used near term, there may be significant respiratory depression of the newborn.[6] The risk categorization changes to a D if used in high doses or at term. Reports on morphine excretion in the breast milk have been variable; however, there is one report of an infant receiving 0.8% to 12% of the maternal dose.[9] There were no short-term adverse effects on the infant. The AAP classifies morphine as compatible with breastfeeding.[6]

PROPOFOL

Propofol, a Category B drug, is a hypnotic agent that is commonly used for the induction and maintenance of anesthesia. During the past several years, it has been increasingly used as a sedative agent for endoscopy. There are limited human data on propofol and pregnancy, but on the basis of animal studies, it is considered a low-risk drug in pregnancy. Animal studies have not shown teratogenic effects. Propofol does rapidly cross the placenta and distribute in the fetus with a fetal maternal ratio of 0.7. When given as anesthesia during delivery, there are no differences in Apgar scores between infants exposed and not exposed to propofol. Depression has been seen in the alert state 1 hour but not 4 hours after intrauterine exposure at delivery. Overall, it is felt to be safe as an anesthetic agent during endoscopy. Due to potentially deeper levels of sedation that may occur with propofol, particular attention should be paid to maintaining adequate maternal oxygen levels. Propofol is excreted into breast milk. The highest levels are 4 to 5 hours after administration.[10] The amounts received in breast milk are much lower than the amounts that are received through placental transfer. It is probably not necessary but reasonable to pump and dump breast milk at 4 to 5 hours postprocedure before resuming breastfeeding.

MIDAZOLAM

Benzodiazepines are classified as Category D medications. Diazepam crosses the placenta and accumulates in the fetal circulation. Midazolam does cross the placenta but more slowly than diazepam and is not concentrated in the fetal circulation. In mice, diazepam exposure has been associated with cleft lip and cleft palate. Midazolam has not been shown to cause similar congenital abnormalities. There is a potential for neonatal respiratory depression in all benzodiazepines. This class of drugs should be used with caution in the pregnant patient and only if the alternative sedative agent is insufficient.[11] Midazolam is excreted into breast milk but is undetectable within 4 hours after a single dose of medication. Nursing should be withheld for at least 4 hours, and consideration should be made of pumping and dumping the first milk produced during this period of time. The AAP lists midazolam as a drug with unknown effects on nursing, but there may be some concern.

REVERSAL AGENTS

NALOXONE

Naloxone, a Category B drug, is a narcotic antagonist that is used during endoscopy to reverse the effects of narcotic analgesics in the event of oversedation. It does cross the placenta and appears in the fetal circulation within several minutes. There have been no reports of fetal damage in animals. Late in gestation, exposure to naloxone causes increase in fetal heart rate accelerations, body movement, and breathing likely due to reversal of the effects of fetal endorphins.[6] It should not be administered to women who are narcotic addicts due to precipitation of opiate withdrawal syndrome in the mother and the infant.[12] Care should be taken with the initial sedation so that naloxone does not have to be used, but if it is needed, then it should be used in small amounts and titrated to effect. Patients should be monitored and supported with oxygen until the effects of the narcotic have worn off and the patient can independently maintain adequate oxygenation. There are no data available on breastfeeding.

FLUMAZENIL

Flumazenil (Category B) reverses the central nervous system effects of benzodiazepines. There are very few data regarding use in pregnancy. It is not known whether there is placental transfer to the fetus; however, the short elimination half-life likely limits the exposure. There have been embryocidal effects reported in rabbits at 200 times the maximum recommended dose.[6] In the case of benzodiazepine overdose, the maternal benefit outweighs the risk to the fetus; however, the situation can be avoided by careful titration of benzodiazepines during endoscopy.

ADJUNCTIVE AGENTS

SIMETHICONE

Simethicone, a Category C drug, is used during endoscopy to aid in visualization of the mucosa. It is a nonabsorbable silicone product that is commonly used as an antiflatulent. There are no reports of congenital defects associated with the use of simethicone. Due to the lack of human and animal data, it is categorized as a C drug during pregnancy; however, it is felt to be relatively safe for the fetus. With the limited exposure during endoscopy, there is no contraindication to its use.[6] There is no contraindication during breastfeeding due to the nonabsorbable nature of the drug.

GLUCAGON

Glucagon (Category B) is commonly used as an antispasmodic during ERCPs. It is a single-chain polypeptide that is identical to human glucagon with a very short elimination half-life (8 to 18 minutes). Glucagon does not cross the placenta in humans or sheep. The risks to the fetus are very low. There are no lactation studies with glucagon; however, due to its short elimination half-life, it is unlikely to be excreted in the milk. If a small amount does get into the milk and is ingested by the nursing infant, it will be rapidly broken down into fragments in the stomach of the infant. It is compatible with breastfeeding.[6]

LIDOCAINE

Lidocaine (Category B) is used as a topical anesthetic during upper gastroenterologic procedures. It rapidly crosses the placenta to the fetus, with detectable levels in the fetal circulation within 1 to 2 minutes after administration intravenously. Less is clear after topical therapy. Lidocaine has not been associated with fetal malformations in humans during the first trimester.[12] Parenteral lidocaine at birth may lead to detectable levels in the newborn that has led to infant central nervous system depression and bradycardia.[6] These levels are much higher than would be expected with topical lidocaine administration. Topical lidocaine is considered safe during pregnancy, although it is recommended that the patient spit out residual lidocaine after gargling.[12] Small amounts of lidocaine do enter the breast milk when large doses are given parenterally. The risk of exposure to lidocaine in breast milk is thought to be very low and is considered compatible with breastfeeding by the AAP.[6]

COLON PREP SOLUTIONS

Colon cleansing products have not been studied in pregnancy. In the general population, PEG electrolyte solutions (Category C) are considered the safest for preparing the colon for a colonoscopy.[13] Magnesium citrate may cause electrolyte disturbances in selected patients. Hyperphosphatemia and renal failure have been described with the use of sodium phosphate-based products.[13] In the pregnant patient, if a colon prep is needed, a PEG-based prep should be used with attention to maintaining the hydration of the patient. For patients undergoing a flexible sigmoidoscopy, consideration of colon preparation with a tap water enema should be made.

SPECIAL CONSIDERATIONS

ELECTROCAUTERY

Electrocautery is used during gastrointestinal endoscopy for a variety of indications, including polypectomy and sphincterotomy. It has been used safely in pregnant patients; however, amniotic fluid has been shown to conduct an electrical current, and precautions must be taken. When possible, postpone polypectomy for an elective date after delivery. The external grounding pad should not be placed so that the uterus is between the electrical device and the grounding pad. Where possible, bipolar current should be used.[11]

ENDOSCOPIC RETROGRADE CHOLANGIOPANCREATOGRAPHY

Endoscopic retrograde cholangiopancreatography (ERCP) can be performed safely during pregnancy, but requires a multidisciplinary approach, and a therapeutic intervention should be clearly indicated and documented.[14] The most common reason for ERCP intervention is choledocholithiasis. Diagnostic ERCP is typically not required. MRCP, abdominal ultrasound, and endoscopic ultrasound can all be used to evaluate the biliary system. ERCP is reserved for therapeutic maneuvers. The modifications that are incorporated into the standard ERCP include standard maternal monitoring, placement of the patient in the left lateral recumbent position to avoid decreased uterine blood flow, and radiation shielding to protect the fetus. Shielding should be above and below the patient, covering the abdomen and pelvis. The sides of the abdomen should be covered with lead shielding.[15] There should be limited fluoroscopy time to protect radiation exposure to the fetus. As an alternative to standard ERCP with fluoroscopy to guide therapy in the bile duct, use of a choledochoscope (SpyGlass, Boston Scientific, Natick, MA) and endoscopic ultrasound (EUS) has been reported for nonfluoroscopic approach to stone therapy.[16]

PERCUTANEOUS ENDOSCOPIC GASTROSTOMY

Percutaneous endoscopic gastrostomy (PEG) has a potentially important role for nutritional support during pregnancy. Coma and severe hyperemesis gravidarum are the 2 most common indications for PEG placement. PEG placement in the third trimester is challenging but possible.[17] The special considerations for PEG placement during pregnancy include the following:

- Ultrasound to identify the dome of the uterus. This should be marked on the patient prior to the procedure.

- Patient should be placed with a wedge under the pelvis (see previous, pelvic tilt) to avoid compression of the vena cava by the gravid uterus. This is preferred to having the patient completely supine as is done for PEG placement in the nongravid patient.

- Monitoring should be performed as above for routine endoscopic procedures in the pregnant patient.

- Preprocedure antibiotics that are safe in pregnancy include penicillins, cephalosporins, and erythromycin (except estolate).[3]

Overall, endoscopy can be performed safely in pregnancy, with appropriate attention to the changes that occur physiologically in the mother during the course of pregnancy and to the growing embryo/fetus. Issues related to endoscopy in the breastfeeding mother take into consideration exposure of the breastfeeding infant to medications that are excreted into breast milk.

REFERENCES

1. Capell M. Sedation and analgesia for gastrointestinal endoscopy during pregnancy. *Gastrointest Endosc Clin North Am.* 2006;16(1):1-31.
2. Cappell M. Endoscopy in pregnancy: risks versus benefits. *Nat Clin Pract Gastroenterol Hepatol.* 2005;2(9):376-377.
3. Qureshi WA, Rajan E, Adler DG, et al. ASGE Guideline: Guidelines for endoscopy in pregnant and lactating women. *Gastrointest Endosc.* 2005;61(3):357-362.
4. ACOG Committee on Obstetric Practice. ACOG Committee Opinion No. 474: nonobstetric surgery during pregnancy. *Obstet Gynecol.* 2011;117(2, pt 1):420-421.
5. Cheek TG, Baird E. Anesthesia for nonobstetric surgery: maternal and fetal considerations. *Clin Obstet Gynecol.* 2009;52(4):535-545.
6. Briggs G, Freeman R, Yaffe S. *Drugs in Pregnancy and Lactation: A Reference Guide to Fetal and Neonatal Risk.* Philadelphia, PA: Lippincott, Williams and Wilkins; 2008.
7. Lindemann R. Respiratory muscle rigidity in a preterm infant after use of fentanyl during Caesarean section. *Eur J Pediatr.* 1998;157(12):1012-1013.
8. Steer PL, Biddle CJ, Marley WS, et al. Concentration of fentanyl in colostrum after an analgesic dose. *Can J Anaesth.* 1992;39(3):231-235.

9. Robieux I, Koren G, Vandenbergh H, Schneiderman J. Morphine excretion in breast milk and resultant exposure of a nursing infant. *J Toxicol Clin Toxicol.* 1990;28(3):365-370.

10. Dalland P, Crockshott ID, Lirzin JD, et al. Intravenous propofol during cesarean section: Placental transfer, concentrations in breast milk and neonatal effects: a preliminary study. *Anesthesiology* 1989;71(6):827-834.

11. Gilinsky NH, Muthunayagam N. Gastrointestinal endoscopy in pregnant and lactating women: emerging standard of care to guide decision-making. *Obstet Gynecol Survey.* 2006;61(12):791-799.

12. Cappell M. Sedation and analgesia for gastrointestinal endoscopy during pregnancy. *Gastrointest Endosc Clin North Am.* 2006;16(1):1-31.

13. Nyberg C, Hendel J, Nielson O. The safety of osmotically acting cathartics in colonic cleansing. *Nat Rev Gastroenterol Hepatol.* 2010;7(10):557-564.

14. Menees S, Elta G. Endoscopic retrograde cholangiopancreatography during pregnancy. *Gastrointest Endosc Clin N Am.* 2006;16(1):41-57.

15. Tang SJ, Mayo MJ, Rodriguez-Frias E, et al. Safety and utility of ERCP during pregnancy. *Gastrointest Endosc.* 2009;69(3, pt 1):453-461.

16. Girotra M, Jani N. Role of endoscopic ultrasound/SpyScope in diagnosis and treatment of choledocholithiasis in pregnancy. *World J Gastroenterol.* 2010;16(28):3601-3602.

17. Senadhi V, Chaudhary J, Dutta S. Percutaneous endoscopic gastrostomy placement during pregnancy in the critical care setting. *Endoscopy.* 2010;42(suppl 2):E358-E359.

9

Surgical Management of the Pregnant Patient

Megan Quintana, MD and Reza Rahbar, MD

Surgical management of the pregnant patient differs in several ways. Pregnancy induces a variety of chemical, hormonal, and mechanical changes that must be factored into the evaluation and treatment of these patients. Often, signs and symptoms of the pregnant patient presenting with GI disorders can be very similar to signs and symptoms of normal pregnancy. Delays in diagnosis and treatment with the misconception that the fetus could be injured may actually lead to unfavorable outcomes. The pregnant patient requires a multidisciplinary approach to care that involves the surgeon, obstetrician, radiologist, and anesthesiologist. In treating a pregnant woman, there are 2 patients to think about, and the physician has responsibility to both. In general, the mother's care will take precedence over the fetus, but appropriate treatment of the mother will usually benefit the fetus as well. About 0.5% to 1% of all pregnant women will require surgery. Fortunately, complications related to nonobstetric surgery are relatively uncommon, occurring in only 1% to 2% of pregnancies.[1] Patient outcomes are best when general anesthesia is postponed until the second trimester when organogenesis is complete, and elective procedures are postponed until after birth.

Isaacs KL, Long MD.
GI and Liver Disease During Pregnancy:
A Practical Approach (pp. 133-152).
© 2013 Taylor & Francis Group

INITIAL MANAGEMENT OF THE PREGNANT PATIENT WITH AN ACUTE ABDOMEN

Management of any pregnant patient presenting with an acute abdomen should begin with a thorough history and physical exam. Important information to obtain includes historical aspects of the pregnancy, current trimester, expected delivery date, and the presence of pregnancy-related complications. An obstetrics consult is appropriate as they can often aid in the decision-making process. Initial management should also include supplemental oxygen, placement of a large-bore IV line for fluid and/or blood administration, and an initial set of labs including a basic metabolic panel, complete blood count, and urinalysis. If the pregnancy is beyond the 24th week, a fetal monitor should be placed.[2] It is important to keep radiographic studies to a minimum. Ultrasonography can be employed. This may not give useful information regarding maternal pathology in the presence of a gravid uterus, but it can also be used to evaluate the fetus.

KEY POINTS

- Initial management of a pregnant patient with an acute abdomen includes the following:
  - ∞ History and physical
  - ∞ Obstetrics consult
  - ∞ Large-bore IV access
  - ∞ Laboratory evaluation
  - ∞ Fetal monitoring
  - ∞ Ultrasound as appropriate

The acute abdomen needs to be addressed immediately, but less acute problems should take into account the stage of pregnancy. The risk of spontaneous abortion is highest during the first trimester. The optimal time for elective surgery is during the second trimester because the uterus is smaller at that time than it is in the third trimester, and because the fetus can be maintained in a relatively stable condition during the administration of general anesthesia.[1]

ACUTE SURGICAL PROBLEMS

TRAUMA

Trauma is believed to occur in approximately 6% to 7% of gestations.[3] Indeed, by some estimates, it may complicate as many as 1 in 12 pregnancies.[4] Trauma remains the leading cause of maternal death, accounting for 46.3% of deaths during pregnancy.[5] Homicide continues to be the most common cause of traumatic maternal death, followed by motor vehicle accident, accidental injury, and suicide.[6] With increased severity of injury to the mother, the danger to the fetus is also increased. Changes during pregnancy may also alter resuscitation of the pregnant patient. Due to the amount of cardiac output that the uterus requires, a uterine injury can lead to massive hemorrhage very quickly. In general, blunt injury is less commonly associated with direct fetal injury given the protection afforded by the gravid uterus. Penetrating injury can pose a more direct risk to the fetus. As pregnancy progresses, the fetus is less protected by the pelvis and more at risk for any type of injury.

Management of the pregnant trauma patient is very similar to management of the nonpregnant trauma patient and always begins with the ABCs (airway, breathing, and circulation). The priority should always remain with the mother, as stabilizing and resuscitating the mother will generally stabilize and support the fetus. Common pitfalls in the resuscitation of the pregnant trauma patient include the following:

- Hypovolemia can be masked due to the expansion of blood volume and increase in cardiac output that is physiologically normal with pregnancy.

- Tachycardia and hypotension may not be accurate indicators of hypovolemia.

- Expanded intravascular blood volume can change the amount of replacement fluid required for resuscitation.

- When pregnancy is greater than 20 weeks, lying supine can cause aortocaval compression by the gravid uterus, leading to hypotension and hypoperfusion.

Radiographs that are crucial for decisions regarding management should be obtained as needed. Ultrasonography can be useful in pregnant trauma patients as it is also useful in assessing the nonpregnant abdomen after trauma. Fetal monitoring may also be a helpful adjunct in assessing the patient once the mother is stabilized. Again, maternal resuscitation maintains priority, and this will most often also benefit the fetus.

APPENDICITIS

Appendicitis is the most common surgical emergency in the pregnant patient. It occurs once in every 1500 to 2000 pregnancies, with approximate equal frequency in each trimester.[7] This condition is considered a surgical emergency. Delayed diagnosis and treatment puts the patient at risk for perforated appendicitis, and perforation is the number one surgical cause of fetal loss during pregnancy.[8] Perforation can lead to a 20% to 25% rate of fetal loss and a 4% maternal mortality, whereas uncomplicated acute appendicitis only results in a fetal mortality of less than 5%.[9]

Diagnosis of Appendicitis
History and Physical Examination

The risk of developing appendicitis is the same in pregnant women and nonpregnant women. Signs and symptoms include nausea, vomiting, anorexia, and periumbilical pain that migrates to the location of the inflamed appendix. Diagnosis can therefore be very difficult as these symptoms commonly mimic many GI disorders in general, and even physiologic changes in uncomplicated pregnancy. In addition, the location of the appendix and its associated pain will change throughout pregnancy, making the location of pain and tenderness misleading at times. After the fifth month of pregnancy, the appendix shifts from the right lower quadrant superiorly above the right iliac crest, and the tip is often rotated medially due to the gravid uterus. Localized tenderness is a less reliable sign as distention of the abdomen lifts the peritoneum away from the area of inflammation and abdominal tenderness is more generalized. However, nearly all patients with appendicitis develop right-sided abdominal pain and tenderness, and this remains a more reliable symptom of appendicitis during pregnancy. Pain can be differentiated from adnexal or uterine pain with the help of the Adler sign: if the point of maximal tenderness shifts medially with repositioning on the left lateral side, the etiology is generally adnexal or uterine rather than appendiceal.[10] Other signs, such as guarding and rebound tenderness, are only present in about 70% of patients and less commonly in the third trimester given the laxity of abdominal musculature.[8] Fever is not a common finding in pregnant patients with appendicitis. Laboratory values can be misleading in that pregnancy can cause a leukocytosis as high as 15,000 leukocytes/ mm^3 in the absence of any source of infection.[11] The white cell differential is more useful than the absolute count; increased levels of band cells or immature forms suggest that the leukocytosis may be secondary to an infectious process. A urinalysis is necessary to rule out a urinary tract infection. Urinalysis is abnormal with pyuria or hematuria in as many as 20% of patients with appendicitis as a result of extraluminal irritation of the ureter by the inflamed appendix.[12]

KEY POINTS

• Symptoms of appendicitis can be nonspecific
  ∞ Nausea and vomiting
  ∞ Anorexia
  ∞ Periumbilical pain
• Classic symptoms of appendicitis may not be present
  ∞ Guarding and rebound may not be present due to laxity of abdominal musculature
  ∞ Fever is not as common
• Site of appendix can be rotated by gravid uterus
• Laboratory values such as leukocytosis can be present due to pregnancy alone

Diagnostic Imaging

With various imaging modalities available, choosing the ideal diagnostic imaging resource can pose a challenge. Diagnostic radiology should be employed deliberately and judiciously. Ultrasonography of the lower abdomen or transvaginal ultrasonography can be used without much risk to the fetus. This may be able to locate an inflamed appendix and look for a periappendiceal abscess. It can also distinguish other causes of abdominal pain, such as an ovarian cyst. At times, history, clinical exam, and ultrasound are sufficient to establish the diagnosis of appendicitis.[13,14] However, it can also be equivocal, necessitating further imaging. CT is more precise than ultrasonography in the diagnosis of appendicitis. It has a diagnostic accuracy rate for acute appendicitis of 93% to 98%.[15] Use of intravenous and oral/rectal contrast media and thin cuts optimizes this study. The CT can show the appendix and periappendiceal area with a good amount of detail and can also be an excellent imaging tool for differentiating appendicitis from most acute gynecologic conditions that might produce similar symptoms to appendicitis in the pregnant woman. Disadvantages of CT include possible iodinated contrast media allergy, renal injury due to contrast, and exposure to ionizing radiation, which can be harmful to the fetus. MRI is another viable option in the imaging of pregnant patients and is helpful in diagnosing acute appendicitis in special patient populations, such as children and pregnant women. Because MRI does not expose the fetus to radiation and is known to be safe overall in the setting of pregnancy, it has become an increasingly attractive diagnostic imaging modality for identifying intra-abdominal pathology in the pregnant patient. Recent studies show that MRI is just as accurate as CT in diagnosing pathologies such as appendicitis and is a safer alternative to the radiation of CT scans, especially during gestation.[16] In one small series, MRI had an overall sensitivity of 100%, a specificity of 93.6%, and an accuracy of 94.0% in the evaluation of potential acute appendicitis.[17] Its negative predictive value was 100%. These results suggest that MRI is an excellent tool for excluding acute appendicitis in pregnant women with acute abdominal pain whose appendices cannot be visualized by means of ultrasonography.[17]

Differential Diagnosis of Right Lower Quadrant Pain

The differential diagnosis of a pregnant woman with right lower quadrant pain and concern for appendicitis can be fairly expansive. The condition most commonly confused with appendicitis is pyelonephritis, which occurs in 1% to 2% of pregnant women. Because of the mechanical effects of the gravid uterus on the ureter, pyelonephritis is more common in pregnant women. The 2 diseases may present extremely similar clinical pictures, especially when pyelonephritis occurs on the right side. Nephrolithiasis can also be mistaken for appendicitis. Right lower quadrant pain during early pregnancy may also represent ectopic implantation. Often with an ectopic pregnancy, there is some degree of vaginal bleeding or spotting. This may help distinguish an ectopic pregnancy from a problem with the appendix. Abdominal or pelvic pain as well as cervical motion tenderness is present, and a mass is often appreciated on pelvic exam. A serum human chorionic gonadotropin (hCG) assay should be performed as well as a transvaginal ultrasound. If the serum hCG level is greater than 2000 IU/L and an intrauterine gestational sac is not visualized by ultrasound, these indicate emergent intervention for ectopic implantation rather than appendicitis. Torsion of an ovary or an ovarian cyst may also be difficult to distinguish from appendicitis.[18] Transvaginal ultrasound can frequently detect the cyst. The differential diagnosis should also include mesenteric adenitis, inflammatory bowel disease, cholecystitis, adhesions, and other problems of gynecologic etiology. For a complete discussion of the differential diagnosis of abdominal pain, see Chapter 4.

Management of Appendicitis

Immediate surgical intervention is recommended once the diagnosis of appendicitis is suspected or confirmed despite what stage the pregnancy has reached.[19] There is no role for nonoperative management with this pathology. Diagnostic laparoscopy can be used in cases where the diagnosis is not completely clear. Given the danger of a perforated appendix to both mother and fetus, a higher rate of negative appendectomy may be acceptable in the pregnant patient. There exists a small risk of fetal loss, but much less so than if there is a delay in treatment. Pregnant patients undergoing surgery for appendicitis should receive perioperative antibiotics such as a cephalosporin, and anaerobic coverage (Table 9-1). Laparoscopy can be performed safely in the first 2 trimesters but becomes more difficult as the uterus reaches a size greater than the umbilicus.[20] In an open operation, the incision is typically placed over the site of maximal tenderness. It is crucial not to place retractors medially against the uterus as this can cause uterine irritability and onset of labor.[21] If rupture or perforation is suspected, it is appropriate to use a midline incision, and skin is left open postoperatively to avoid wound infections. It is appropriate to treat a contained appendiceal abscess with percutaneous drainage and antibiotics. An interval appendectomy can then be performed later as long as the patient improves with initial management. The premature delivery rate for pregnant women undergoing appendectomy ranges from 13% to 22%.[7]

Table 9-1

Medications Used in the Pregnant Patient Prior to Surgery

	FDA Pregnancy Category*	Pregnancy Comment
Antibiotics		
Cephalosporin (1st through 4th generation)	B	Low risk
Ampicillin	B	Low risk
Metronidazole	B	Low risk; avoid in first trimester
Piperacillin/ tazobactam	B	Low risk
Analgesics		
Meperidine	B	Crosses blood-brain barrier of fetus more slowly than morphine Do not use repetitive high doses Do not use high doses at term
Morphine	C	No congenital abnormalities when used in first trimester Risk in third trimester or in high doses at term
Fentanyl	C	Rapid first-pass clearance Avoid high doses Less respiratory depression of infant at term than with meperidine

Adapted from Mahadevan U, Kane S. American Gastroenterological Association Institute medical position statement on the use of gastrointestinal medications in pregnancy. *Gastroenterology.* 2006;131(1):278-282.

*See Appendix for discussion of FDA pregnancy categories.

KEY POINTS
• Surgical management of appendicitis includes the following: ∞ Immediate surgical intervention once diagnosis is made.   ∞ Diagnostic laparoscopy can be performed when uncertain.   ∞ In an open procedure, it is crucial not to place retractors medially against the uterus as this can cause uterine irritability and onset of labor.   ∞ If a rupture or perforation is suspected, skin can be left open postoperatively to avoid wound infections.   ∞ Rate of premature delivery for women undergoing appendectomy ranges from 13% to 22%.

URGENT SURGICAL PROBLEMS

BILIARY TRACT DISEASES

Biliary tract diseases are the second most common GI disorder requiring surgery during pregnancy.[9] Gallstones form in about 7% of nulliparous women but in 19% of women with multiple pregnancies.[22] The incidence of gallstone disease in pregnant women ranges from 3.3% to 12.2% and increases with gestational age.[23] Pregnant women are already at a predisposition for gallstones given delayed GI motility and biliary stasis. Symptomatic gallstone disease is also common during pregnancy and describes right upper quadrant pain without signs and symptoms of associated inflammation or infection.

Pathophysiology of Gallstone Disease

Gallstone disease is a result of cholesterol supersaturation and biliary stasis, both of which are promoted by pregnancy.[24] The elevation of estrogen levels during pregnancy increases cholesterol secretion by the liver. Estrogen enhances hepatic cholesterol uptake, increases cholesterol synthesis, and inhibits catabolism of cholesterol to bile acids. High concentrations of cholesterol in the bile overwhelm the solubilizing ability of bile salts, with the result that cholesterol stones form.[25] Elevated progesterone levels lead to bile stasis and decreased gallbladder contraction. Progesterone also causes incomplete emptying of the gallbladder after stimulation by cholecystokinin (CCK).[26] The mechanisms are not fully understood, but it is presumed that progesterone may decrease gallbladder reactivity to CCK.[27] The decrease in small-bowel motility that occurs due to progesterone elevation may alter enterohepatic circulation and decrease bile acid return to the liver as well.[28] The balance of bile salts and cholesterol is further altered in such a way as to favor cholesterol supersaturation and stone formation. Pregnancy also alters the pool of bile acids. The decreased percentage of chenodeoxycholic acid and the increased percentage of cholic acid during pregnancy also promote stone formation.

Management of Gallstone Disease

The recommended management of uncomplicated biliary colic during pregnancy is medical management. Signs and symptoms of uncomplicated gallstone disease are similar among pregnant and nonpregnant women and mainly include right upper quadrant or epigastric pain associated with nausea, vomiting, and anorexia. Surgery for symptomatic gallstone disease should be avoided until after pregnancy if possible. However, 1 to 8 of 10,000 pregnant women will suffer from acute cholecystitis, and these women may require surgical intervention. Invasive procedures are better tolerated when performed during the second trimester.[29] Maternal and fetal complications are uncommon, and the risk of fetal demise or preterm delivery is minimized when elective procedures are done in the second trimester. Risks of delayed intervention, however, include infection, pancreatitis, and gallbladder rupture. These can lead to increased rates of fetal mortality.[30] Cholecystectomy during pregnancy should be reserved for recurrent biliary colic or complications from biliary tract disease. Complications such as cholecystitis, gallstone pancreatitis, or symptoms of recurrent biliary colic compromising the health of mother or fetus (intractable nausea, maternal weight loss, fetal growth retardation) are indications for cholecystectomy.

KEY POINTS
• Uncomplicated biliary colic should be medically managed with avoidance of surgery if possible. • Complicated gallstone disease requires surgery. • Surgery for gallstone disease should be performed during the second trimester if possible.

Cholecystitis

Gallstone disease causes acute cholecystitis in only 0.05% to 0.08% of births.[31] Clinical symptoms of cholecystitis consist of the same epigastric or right upper quadrant pain, nausea, and vomiting and also may include fever. Physical findings include tenderness in the right upper quadrant and, occasionally, Murphy's sign. Elevated liver function test results indicate that complicated biliary tract disease or choledocholithiasis is likely; however, elevated alkaline phosphatase levels are also seen in normal pregnancies and, thus, are diagnostically less helpful.

Diagnostic Imaging

Ultrasound can again be a helpful diagnostic tool. Right upper quadrant ultrasound has been shown to be accurate 97% of the time in diagnosing gallstones and biliary ductal dilatation.[32] Ultrasonographic signs of acute cholecystitis remain similar to nonpregnant patients and include gallbladder wall thickening, pericholecystic fluid, biliary ductal dilatation, and an ultrasonographic-positive Murphy's sign.[33] Radionuclide scans introduce the risk of fetal exposure to radiation. This risk almost always outweighs the potential value of any information to be gained from such a scan.

Differential Diagnosis

Differential diagnosis of right upper quadrant pain includes cholecystitis, appendicitis, pyelonephritis, nephrolithiasis, acute pancreatitis, myocardial infarction, gastroesophageal reflux disease, peptic ulcer disease, hepatitis, and hepatic liver abscess. Significant hepatic syndromes can occur during pregnancy, such as intrahepatic cholestasis of pregnancy, acute fatty liver of pregnancy, infectious hepatitis, the hemolysis, elevated liver enzymes, low platelet count syndrome (HELLP), and eclampsia.[34] For a complete description of the differential diagnosis of abdominal pain, see Chapter 4.

Management of Biliary Tract Disease (Cholelithiasis, Cholecystitis)

Initial management of biliary tract disease including cholelithiasis and cholecystitis in the pregnant patient does not require immediate surgical intervention. Bowel rest should be initiated with antimicrobial therapy and adequate analgesia as required. It is also important to provide adequate intravenous hydration. Serial monitoring of liver enzyme tests and amylase levels is essential during medical management to monitor for worsening or progression of disease. This regimen is successful in 84% of patients.[35] If the patient fails to respond to these measures or continues to have repeated attacks of biliary colic requiring hospitalization, then surgical management becomes an appropriate option. Other indications for surgery include intractable nausea, maternal weight loss, fetal growth retardation, obstructive jaundice, gallstone pancreatitis, or peritonitis. Symptomatic gallstone disease is also an indication for surgical intervention.

Surgical Management: Cholecystectomy

If cholecystectomy is necessary during pregnancy but not urgent, it is best tolerated when deferred to the second trimester if possible. Fetal mortality from a first-trimester cholecystectomy can be as high as 12%,[36] but decreases to less than 5% during second- or third-trimester surgical intervention.[37] The rate of fetal loss decreases through gestation; however, beginning in the third trimester, the risk of preterm labor increases. Laparoscopic cholecystectomy is safe in most pregnant patients. Advantages of a laparoscopic approach include less pain and a quicker recovery. Port sites should be placed to avoid injury to the gravid uterus. End tidal or arterial CO_2 levels should be carefully monitored, as hypercapnia can lead to fetal acidosis. Intraoperative ultrasonography is safe for assessment of the biliary tract. Open common duct exploration can also be performed if choledocholithiasis is suspected.

Interventional Management: Cholecystostomy Tube Placement

Another option that is gaining acceptance in the management of acute cholecystitis is percutaneous drainage via cholecystostomy tube placed under ultrasound guidance. Medical treatment of acute cholecystitis in pregnancy may lead to prolonged management and recurrent hospitalizations, whereas surgical management predisposes the mother and fetus to the inherent risks of surgery and general anesthesia. Percutaneous cholecystostomy has been proven to be an efficacious treatment in critically ill and general surgery patients who are at high risk for surgery, but this technique has not been used routinely as a treatment for acute cholecystitis in pregnancy. Percutaneous cholecystostomy may provide a safe and effective alternative for the palliation of acute cholecystitis in pregnancy until a postpartum cholecystectomy can be performed.[38]

Endoscopic Management of Choledocholithiasis

In patients with choledocholithiasis, intervention should be performed without delay. The common bile duct should be explored by means of ERCP. This uses fluoroscopy, and lead aprons can be used to protect the fetus. In experienced hands, ERCP can be performed in some instances with minimal to no fluoroscopy exposure. ERCP with sphincterotomy successfully addresses choledocholithiasis without increasing fetal mortality or the rate of preterm delivery.[39] Choledocholithiasis with right upper quadrant tenderness, fever, and jaundice (Charcot's triad) suggests cholangitis. The only treatment options for cholangitis when ERCP fails are open cholecystectomy and percutaneous intubation of bile ducts.[40] Further information on endoscopic procedures in pregnancy can be found in Chapter 8.

INTESTINAL OBSTRUCTION

Intestinal obstruction is the third most common nonobstetric reason for laparotomy in pregnant patients. Obstruction is most common in the third trimester. Signs and symptoms are vague and similar to many abdominal and gynecologic pathologies. These include acute abdominal pain, nausea, and vomiting. However, a distinguishing feature is the inability to pass stool or, more importantly, gas per rectum. Causes of intestinal obstruction include adhesions, volvulus, intussusception, internal hernia, or neoplasm, the most common of which being adhesions, which account for 55% of cases. Volvulus accounts for 25% of cases.[41] As the incidence of operative procedures and the average age of the mother at gestation have risen, the likelihood of adhesive obstruction has also increased. This may be further exacerbated by the hypo-motility or dysmotility known to occur during pregnancy.[42] Diagnosis can be confirmed with imaging, such as an acute abdominal film. On x-ray, dilated bowel loops and air-fluid levels can support the diagnosis.

Large-bowel obstruction is less common than small-bowel obstruction, but can be seen more often as pregnancy progresses. The most common cause is cecal or sigmoid volvulus. Volvulus during pregnancy is associated with a 21% to 43% mortality rate.[43] Colonic pseudo-obstruction, or Ogilvie syndrome, has also been reported late in pregnancy or in the early puerperium.[44] Extreme colonic dilatation without anatomic obstruction is apparent, with gas filling the entire length of the colon from cecum to rectum. The danger of cecal perforation is high when the maximum diameter of the cecum exceeds 12 cm.

MANAGEMENT OF INTESTINAL OBSTRUCTION

Management of intestinal obstruction in pregnant patients is similar to nonpregnant patients and includes decompression with a nasogastric tube connected to suction, IV hydration, and timely surgery. Any sign of bowel ischemia or perforation in a pregnant patient with intestinal obstruction should prompt immediate surgical intervention. The need for laparotomy and lysis of adhesions during pregnancy is extremely low; however, when surgical management is necessary, fetal mortality is 26%, and maternal mortality is 5%. With intestinal obstruction, the main concern is ensuring that the diagnosis is not delayed. Accordingly, any pregnant patient presenting with nausea, vomiting, and a history of abdominal surgery should be presumed to have a small-bowel obstruction until proven otherwise.

KEY POINTS

• Management of intestinal obstruction includes the following:
  ∞ Decompression with NG tube to suction
  ∞ Bowel rest
  ∞ IV fluid support
  ∞ Signs of bowel ischemia or perforation should prompt immediate surgical intervention

HEMORRHOIDS

Hemorrhoids are a common complaint of pregnant women, and nearly 10% of obstetric patients have hemorrhoids at some point during pregnancy.[45] While most often managed medically, hemorrhoids can require surgical intervention. It is thought that hemorrhoids are exacerbated by the increased circulating volume in a pregnant woman compounded by compression of the superior rectal veins by the gravid uterus, causing increased venous congestion.[46] Additionally, progesterone has a relaxing effect on the smooth muscle in vein walls. Patients will present with bleeding, hemorrhoidal prolapse, rectal pruritus, and generalized discomfort. Severe pain can be a sign of thrombosed hemorrhoid. It is important to rule out other causes of these symptoms, such as inflammatory bowel disorders, anal fissure, and colorectal or anal cancer if the patient does not respond to appropriate medical therapies for hemorrhoids.

TREATMENT OF HEMORRHOIDS

Treatment is preferably nonoperative, especially during pregnancy. Dietary fiber is recommended, as are stool softeners, increased fluid intake, psyllium, avoidance of straining, warm sitz baths, and topical hemorrhoidal analgesics. Methods to alleviate associated constipation should be employed (see Chapter 5). If the patient is found to have internal hemorrhoids, rubber band ligation is an option that can be performed in the office without general anesthesia. Hemorrhoidectomy is rarely indicated during pregnancy and is usually only required if severely prolapsed hemorrhoids are present or if there is associated ulceration, severe rectal bleeding, fissure or fistula symptoms, and failure to respond to or inability to tolerate nonoperative measures. Acutely thrombosed external hemorrhoids can be treated with incision and clot extraction or excision performed with local anesthetic.[47]

KEY POINTS

- Management of hemorrhoids includes the following:
  - ∞ Medical management should be optimized, with avoidance of surgical management if possible.
  - ∞ Treat associated factors such as constipation.
  - ∞ Surgical interventions are only employed with severely prolapsed hemorrhoids, severe ulceration, rectal bleeding, fissure, or failure to respond to nonoperative measures.

COLORECTAL CANCER

Malignancy of the colon and rectum is extremely rare in pregnant patients, given their age distribution and the fact that colorectal cancer (CRC) is typically found in the 5th and 6th decades of life. With pregnancy, there can be an increase in rectal examinations, allowing for increased detection of rectal carcinoma. This may account for rectal carcinoma being slightly more common in pregnancy. Once again, there is often a delay in diagnosis given the vague, nonspecific nature of symptoms associated with CRC. Additionally, some laboratory markers traditionally associated with malignancy, such as carcinoembryonic antigen (CEA), can be elevated in physiologic pregnancy. Diagnosis relies on digital rectal exam, testing for occult blood per rectum, and flexible sigmoidoscopy, which is a safe option in pregnancy if indicated. Optimal timing of sigmoidoscopy is during the second trimester, if possible (see Chapter 8). Management is similar to that for nonpregnant patients. In the first 20 weeks, patients can undergo colorectal resection without hysterectomy. If CRC is found later in pregnancy, it is best to delay surgery for fetal maturation if possible. Complications of CRC can be dangerous and include hemorrhage, obstruction, and colonic perforation. Tumors below the pelvic brim may make vaginal delivery difficult, and

C-section should be considered in these patients. Current survival data are similar for both pregnant and nonpregnant women with CRC. Chemotherapy poses a significant risk to the fetus, and is therefore not usually recommended until after delivery.

SUMMARY

Surgical management of the pregnant patient differs from that of the nonpregnant patient. There can be important differences in the presentation of the pregnant patient with acute GI disorders, such as appendicitis or cholecystitis. Delays in diagnosis and treatment with the misconception that the fetus could be injured can lead to unfavorable outcomes. Common surgical procedures and associated mortality during pregnancy are shown in Table 9-2. In general, surgical procedures are safe during pregnancy, with increased safety associated with earlier recognition of the GI disorder. For example, the maternal and fetal mortality associated with a routine appendectomy is much lower than that associated with a ruptured appendicitis. Necessary diagnostic studies should be performed to appropriately diagnose and treat the mother. Absolute indications for surgery in a pregnant woman (Table 9-3) should be adhered to in a timely fashion. Often, surgical approaches and intraoperative management can differ for the pregnant patient as well. A multidisciplinary approach is required to ensure appropriate care for both mother and fetus.

REFERENCES

1. Barron WM. The pregnant surgical patient: medical evaluation and management. *Ann Intern Med.* 1984;101:683-691.
2. Brooks DC, Oxford C: The pregnant surgical patient. In: Ashley SW, ed. *ACS Surgery: Principles and Practice.* Philadelphia: American College of Surgeons; 2010.
3. Hoff WS, D'Amelio LF, Tinkoff GH, et al. Maternal predictors of fetal demise in trauma during pregnancy. *Surg Gynecol Obstet.* 1991;172(3):175-180.
4. American College of Obstetricians and Gynecologists. *Educational Bulletin: Obstetric Aspects of Trauma Management.* 1998;251:297-303.
5. Fildes J, Reed L, Jones N, Martin M, Barrett J. Trauma: the leading cause of maternal death. *J Trauma.* 1992;32(5):643-645.
6. Pearlman MD, Tintinalli JE, Lorenz RP. Blunt trauma during pregnancy. *N Engl J Med.* 1990;323(23):1609-1613.

Table 9-2

Common Surgical Procedures and Associated Mortality During Pregnancy

Surgical Procedure	Mortality
Exploratory laparotomy	• Maternal mortality: 5% • Fetal mortality: 26%
Open appendectomy	Routine surgical management: • Maternal mortality: negligible • Fetal mortality: 2% to 8% Ruptured appendicitis: • Maternal mortality: 1% • Fetal mortality: 35%
Laparoscopic cholecystectomy	• Maternal mortality: 0.1% • Fetal mortality during a first trimester cholecystectomy: 12% • Fetal mortality during second or third trimester: <5%
Open cholecystectomy	Similar to rates for laparoscopic cholecystectomy

Table 9-3

Absolute Indications for Surgery in Pregnant Women

- Suspected/confirmed appendicitis
- Perforated or ruptured viscous
- Gallstone disease
  - ∞ Failure of conservative management, recurrent disease, intractable nausea, maternal weight loss, fetal growth retardation, obstructive jaundice, gallstone pancreatitis, or peritonitis
- Hemorrhoids
  - ∞ Severely prolapsed hemorrhoids, severe ulceration of hemorrhoids, severe rectal bleeding, fissure or fistula symptoms, or failure to respond to or inability to tolerate nonoperative measures

7. Al-Mulhim AA. Acute appendicitis in pregnancy. A review of 52 cases. *Int Surg.* 1996;81(3):295-297.

8. Weingold AB. Appendicitis in pregnancy. *Clin Obstet Gynecol.* 1983;26(4):801-809.

9. Visser BC, Glasgow RE, Mulvihill KK, Mulvihill SJ. Safety and timing of nonobstetric abdominal surgery in pregnancy. *Dig Surg.* 2001;18(5):409-417.

10. Firstenberg MS, Malangoni MA. Pregnancy and gastrointestinal disorders: gastrointestinal surgery during pregnancy. *Gastroenterol Clin.* 1998;27(1):73-88.

11. Lavin JP Jr, Polsky SS. Abdominal trauma during pregnancy. *Clin Perinatol.* 1983;10(2):423-438.

12. Tamir IL, Bongard FS, Klein SR. Acute appendicitis in the pregnant patient. *Am J Surg.* 1990;160(6):571-575.

13. Adams DH, Fine C, Brooks DC. High-resolution real-time ultrasonography. A new tool in the diagnosis of acute appendicitis. *Am J Surg.* 1988;155(1):93-97.

14. Anderson JM, Lee TG, Nagel N. Ultrasound diagnosis of nonobstetric disease during pregnancy. *Obstet Gynecol.* 1976;48(3):359-362.

15. Rao PM, Rhea JT, Novelline RA, Mostafavi AA, McCabe CJ. Effect of computed tomography of the appendix on treatment of patients and use of hospital resources. *N Engl J Med.* 1998;338(3):141-146.

16. Israel GM, Malguria N, McCarthy S, Copel J, Weinreb J. MRI vs. ultrasound for suspected appendicitis during pregnancy. *J Magn Reson Imaging.* 2008;28(2):428-433.

17. Pedrosa I, Levine D, Eyvazzadeh AD. Siewert B, Ngo L, Rofsky NM. MR imaging evaluation of acute appendicitis in pregnancy. *Radiology.* 2006;238(3):891-899.

18. Horowitz MD, Gomez GA, Santiesteban R, Burkett G. Acute appendicitis during pregnancy: diagnosis and management. *Arch Surg.* 1985;120(12):1362-1367.

19. McComb P, Laimon H. Appendicitis complicating pregnancy. *Can J Surg.* 1980;23(1):92-94.

20. Firstenberg MS, Malangoni MA. Gastrointestinal surgery during pregnancy. *Gastroenterol Clin North Am.* 1998;27(1):73-88.

21. Parangi S, Levine D, Henry A, Isakovich N, Pories S. Surgical gastrointestinal disorders during pregnancy. Am J Surg. 2007 Feb;193(2):223-232.

22. Gilat T, Konikoff F. Pregnancy and the biliary tract. *Can J Gastroenterol.* 2000;14(suppl D):55D-59D.

23. Valdivieso V, Covarrubias C, Siegel F, Cruz F. Pregnancy and cholelithiasis: pathogenesis and natural course of gallstones diagnosed in early puerperium. *Hepatology.* 1993;17(1):1-4.

24. Yates MR, Baron TH. Biliary tract disease in pregnancy. *Clin Liver Dis.* 1999;3:1.

25. Everson GT, McKinley C, Kern F Jr. Mechanisms of gallstone formation in women: effects of exogenous estrogen (Premarin) and dietary cholesterol on hepatic lipid metabolism. *J Clin Invest.* 1991;87(1):237-246.

26. Tierney S, Nakeeb A, Wong O, et al. Progesterone alters biliary flow dynamics. *Ann Surg.* 1999;229(2):2.

27. Ryan JP. Effect of pregnancy on gallbladder contractility in guinea pig. *Gastroenterology.* 1984;87(3):674-678.
28. Kern F Jr, Everson GT, DeMark B, et al. Biliary lipids, bile acids, and gallbladder function in the human female: effects of pregnancy and the ovulatory cycle. *J Clin Invest.* 1981;68(5):1229-1242.
29. Kammerer WS. Nonobstetric surgery in pregnancy. *Med Clin North Am.* 1987;71(3):551-560.
30. Curet MJ, Allen D, Josloff RK, et al. Laparoscopy during pregnancy. *Arch Surg.* 1996;131(5):546-550.
31. Ramin KD, Ramsey PS. Medical complications of pregnancy: disease of the gall bladder and pancreas in pregnancy. *Obstet Gynecol Clin.* 2001;28(3):571-580.
32. Reece EA, Assimakopoulos E, Zheng XZ, Hagay Z, Hobbins JC. The safety of obstetric ultrasonography: concern for the fetus. *Obstet Gynecol.* 1990;76(1):139-146.
33. Woodhouse DR, Haylen B. Gallbladder disease complicating pregnancy. *Aust NZ J Obstet Gynaecol.* 1985;25(3):233-237.
34. Bynum TE. Hepatic and gastrointestinal disorders in pregnancy. *Med Clin North Am.* 1977;61(1):129-138.
35. Landers D, Carmona R, Crombleholme W, Lim R. Acute cholecystitis in pregnancy. *Obstet Gynecol.* 1987;69(1):131-133.
36. McKellar DP, Anderson CT, Boynton CJ. Cholecystectomy during pregnancy without fetal loss. *Surg Obstet Gynecol.* 1992;174:465.
37. Printen KJ, Ott RA. Cholecystectomy during pregnancy. *Am Surg.* 1978;44(7):432-434.
38. Allmendinger N, Hallisey MJ, Ohki SK, Straub JJ. Percutaneous cholecystostomy treatment of acute cholecystitis in pregnancy. *Obstet Gynecol.* 1995;86(4, pt 2):653-654.
39. Baillie J, Cairns SR, Putman WS. Endoscopic management of choledocholithiasis during pregnancy. *Surg Gynecol Obstet.* 1990;171(1):1-4.
40. Strasberg SM. Laparoscopic biliary surgery. *Gastroenterol Clin.* 1999;28(1):117-132.
41. Perdue PW, Johnson HW, Stafford PW. Intestinal obstruction complicating pregnancy. *Am J Surg.* 1992;164(4):384-388.
42. Milne B, Johnstone MS. Intestinal obstruction in pregnancy. *Scott Med J.* 1979;24(1):80-82.
43. Ballantyne GH. Review of sigmoid volvulus: clinical patterns and pathogenesis. *Dis Colon Rectum.* 1985;25(8):823-830.
44. Shaxted EJ, Jukes R. Pseudo-obstruction of the bowel in pregnancy: case reports. *Br J Obstet Gynaecol.* 1979;86(5):411-413.
45. Medich DS, Fazio VW. Hemorrhoids, anal fissure and carcinoma of the colon rectum and anus during pregnancy. *Surg Clin North Am.* 1995;75(1):77-88.
46. Hulme-Moir M, Bartolo DC. Hemorrhoids. *Gastroenterol Clin North Am.* 2001;30(1):183-197.
47. Saleeby RG Jr, Rosen L, Stasik JJ, Riether RD, Sheets J, Khubchandani IT. Hemorrhoidectomy during pregnancy: risk or relief? *Dis Colon Rectum.* 1991;34(3):260-261.

10

Pancreatitis and Biliary Issues

Patricia D. Jones, MD and Lisa M. Gangarosa, MD

PANCREATITIS

EPIDEMIOLOGY

Pancreatitis in pregnancy is a rare entity. Historically, incidence was reported as 1 in 12,000 pregnancies.[1-4] However, in recent retrospective analyses, incidence was found to vary from 1 in 1000 to 1 in 3000 cases.[1,4-7] This increase in incidence is likely related to several factors, the most important being the ability to diagnose pancreatitis by serum amylase and lipase levels, which was not possible in the 1970s.[2] In general, pancreatitis occurs in nulliparous women one-third of the time and in multiparous women two-thirds of the time.[1] Most cases of pancreatitis in pregnant women occur in the second and third trimesters.[1,5-7] This corresponds directly to the increased incidence of biliary stone disease as gestational age increases. There is no definite racial predominance noted.

Isaacs KL, Long MD.
*GI and Liver Disease During Pregnancy:
A Practical Approach (pp. 153-166).*
© 2013 Taylor & Francis Group

DIAGNOSIS/PRESENTING SIGNS/SYMPTOMS

The presentation of pancreatitis is not different in pregnant women and includes nausea, vomiting, abdominal pain, and occasionally fever. The differential diagnosis of acute pancreatitis includes biliary colic, acute cholecystitis, acute cholangitis, acute fatty liver in pregnancy, HELLP syndrome, acute appendicitis, peptic ulcer disease, and intestinal obstruction. As in nonpregnant patients, the diagnosis of pancreatitis is confirmed by elevated serum amylase and lipase levels that are greater than 3 times the upper limit of normal. Other tests such as bilirubin, alkaline phosphatase, GGT, AST, and ALT should establish whether a biliary source is the cause. In normal pregnancies, alkaline phosphatase is elevated.

MANAGEMENT OF PANCREATITIS

Pancreatitis in pregnancy is managed no differently than pancreatitis in the nonpregnant patient. It is beyond the scope of this chapter to cover this in depth, but several excellent reviews are available.[8-10] The initial management of pancreatitis depends on the severity, which can be determined using the Ranson criteria[11] or Acute Physiology and Chronic Health Evaluation II (APACHE II) score.[12] The mainstay of therapy is aggressive intravenous fluid hydration. In addition, supportive care with antiemetics and analgesia is provided. Early introduction of oral nutrition is preferred when tolerated. In severe pancreatitis, enteral nutrition via a nasojejunal tube may be necessary. Enteral nutrition maintains GI physiology, allowing gut flora to maintain mucosal immunity and prevent bacterial translocation.[13] Parenteral nutrition (TPN) is associated with the risk of infection, metabolic derangements, and hyperlipidemia and should be avoided whenever possible, but may be required in cases of severe or triglyceride-induced pancreatitis. Analgesics commonly used and safe in pregnancy include morphine, fentanyl, and hydromorphone.

Antibiotics should not be used routinely in patients with pancreatitis but should be reserved for patients with superimposed acute cholecystitis, cholangitis, or necrotizing pancreatitis with infection (Table 10-1).

Table 10-1

Medications for Pancreatitis and Biliary Disease During Pregnancy and Breastfeeding

Medication	FDA Pregnancy Category*	Pregnancy Comment	Breastfeeding Comment
Analgesics			
Meperidine	B	Crosses blood-brain barrier of fetus more slowly than MSO4 Do not use repetitive high doses Do not use high doses at term	May be detected up to 24 hours after administration.
Morphine	C	No congenital abnormalities when used in first trimester Risk in third trimester or in high doses at term	Does cross into breast milk—no immediate adverse effects on newborn AAP considers compatible
Fentanyl	C	Rapid first pass clearance Avoid high doses Less respiratory depression of infant at term than with meperidine	At 10 hours, undetectable in breast milk Low oral bioavailability Compatible
Hydro-morphone	C	Teratogenic in animals at 600 times the human dose	Does cross into breast milk with half-life in milk of 10.5 hours Breastfed infant receives 0.67% of the maternal dose-adjusted for body weight

(continued)

Table 10-1 *(continued)*

Medications for Pancreatitis and Biliary Disease During Pregnancy and Breastfeeding

Medication	FDA Pregnancy Category*	Pregnancy Comment	Breastfeeding Comment
Antibiotics*			
Imipenem	C	No teratogenicity in animals	Acceptable for use Maternal doses lead to low levels in breast milk Not expected to cause adverse effects
Meropenem	B	No embryotoxicity or teratogenicity in animal studies	No information available
Piperacillin/ tazobactam	B	No embryotoxicity or teratogenicity in animal studies	Maternal doses lead to low levels in breast milk not expected to cause adverse effects
Ampicillin/ sulbactam	B	No embryotoxicity or teratogenicity in animal studies	Acceptable for use Maternal doses lead to low levels in breast milk not expected to cause adverse effects

(continued)

Table 10-1 *(continued)*

Medications for Pancreatitis and Biliary Disease During Pregnancy and Breastfeeding

Medication	FDA Pregnancy Category*	Pregnancy Comment	Breastfeeding Comment
Sedatives			
Propofol	B	Not teratogenic; short acting but can cross placenta	Amounts in breast milk very small No sedation noted in breast-fed infants
Diazepam	D	Possibly associated with neonatal cleft lip and palate and other congenital abnormalities	Excreted into breast milk For a single dose for procedure, no need to wait if term infant, but mat wait 6 to 8 hours if preterm
Midazolam	D	Transiently depresses neonatal respiration; similar to diazepam; however, no teratogenic effects found	Small amounts excreted into breast milk No waiting period or discarding milk necessary May lead to transient decrease in milk production
Miscellaneous			
Omega-3 fatty acids		Critical for fetal neurodevelopment	Thought to be helpful for brain development

(continued)

Table 10-1 *(continued)*

Medications for Pancreatitis and Biliary Disease During Pregnancy and Breastfeeding

Medication	FDA Pregnancy Category*	Pregnancy Comment	Breastfeeding Comment
Calcitonin	C	Animal studies using synthetic salmon calcitonin have shown a decrease in fetal birth weights when rabbits at doses 14 to 56 times the recommended human dose	Calcitonin is a normal component of human milk, levels are generally found at 40 times that of serum. Likely digested in the infant's GI tract
Fenofibrate	C	Animal studies with doses 7 to 10 times the recommended human dosage based on body surface area (BSA) have demonstrated embryocidal and teratogenic effects (skeletal abnormalities, decreased live births/survival)	No information available

Adapted from Mahadevan U, Kane S. American Gastroenterological Association Institute medical position statement on the use of gastrointestinal medications in pregnancy. *Gastroenterology.* 2006;131(1):278-282.

Note: Prophylactic use of antibiotics not recommended by the American College of Gastroenterology, and the American Gastroenterological Association recommends restricting antibiotic prophylaxis to patients with substantial (>30% of gland) necrosis.

*See Appendix for discussion of FDA pregnancy categories.

FURTHER INVESTIGATION

In all patients with acute pancreatitis, abdominal ultrasound should be performed to evaluate for cholelithiasis. Although CT scan may be used to evaluate the severity of pancreatitis in nonpregnant patients, this should be avoided in the pregnant patient to prevent unnecessary radiation exposure to the developing fetus. If there is no evidence of biliary disease by ultrasound or laboratory testing, calcium and triglyceride levels should be obtained. A thorough history should reveal if alcohol is causative, and serum alcohol levels can be performed if there remains a strong suspicion despite history provided.

CAUSES OF PANCREATITIS

Once diagnosed, care should be taken to determine the etiology of acute pancreatitis as this will potentially affect management. Pancreatitis is caused by gallstones in 60% to 70% of cases.[1-3,5,7] Other etiologies include hypertriglyceridemia, with a frequency reported as 1 in 25,000 cases[14] but accounting for up to 4% of cases in a recent series.[5] Alcohol is often associated with chronic pancreatitis and accounted for up to 12% of cases in this same series.[5] Rare causes include hyperparathyroidism, iatrogenic (post-ERCP for treatment of choledocholithiasis), medication-induced (eg, diuretics, antibiotics, antihypertensives, azathioprine), connective tissue diseases, abdominal surgery, infections, genetic mutations, and blunt abdominal trauma.[3,8] In 16.5% of patients, no cause was identified in a case series.[5]

BILIARY PANCREATITIS

In pregnant patients with gallstone pancreatitis, conservative management alone may be appropriate, depending on the trimester of presentation. If the patient presents in the second trimester, it is generally accepted practice to allow the acute episode of pancreatitis to subside, and then proceed to cholecystectomy. Patients who are treated conservatively have more frequent relapses and subsequent hospitalizations.[2,4,5] The earlier one presents, the more likely he or she will relapse during the remainder of his or her pregnancy. Relapses are often more serious than the initial presentation.[4,6,7] Pregnant women who have elective cholecystectomy are less likely to require emergent surgery and are more likely to deliver at term.[4,5,7,15] Retrospective reviews of case records have demonstrated no increase in fetal or maternal morbidity and mortality when cholecystectomy is performed.[3,4,7,10] There may be a small increase in the incidence of premature contractions surrounding the surgery. However, this is usually managed successfully with tocolysis. In fact, fetal outcomes are better in women treated surgically[3,4,7,10]; however, surgery should be timed for the second trimester after organogenesis is complete, but before the uterus is large enough to obstruct the surgical field.

In the event of cholestasis and ductal dilatation on ultrasound, magnetic resonance cholangiopancreatography (MRCP) or endoscopic ultrasound (EUS) should be performed to evaluate for choledocholithiasis. There is theoretical concern about the safety of MRCP in the first trimester, as radio frequency pulses could lead to heating of fetal tissues, but there is no radiation risk.[3,8] EUS has a positive predictive value of 100% in detecting common bile duct (CBD) stones and may be superior to MRCP; however, it is an endoscopic procedure requiring sedation (see Chapter 8).[8] An ERCP could be performed directly following the EUS using the same sedation if EUS is positive. Diagnostic ERCP is no longer used during pregnancy, but therapeutic ERCP should be performed in the setting of choledocholithiasis or in any case of severe pancreatitis with CBD obstruction (see Chapter 8). ERCP with sphincterotomy protects against recurrent episodes of pancreatitis and complications such as cholangitis, which lead to increased mortality and morbidity.[3] Care should be taken to minimize fetal exposure to radiation. In patients undergoing ERCP with sphincterotomy in one series, there was no increase in adverse fetal outcomes, and there were no recurrences of acute biliary pancreatitis.[6]

KEY POINT

- If a pregnant woman develops complications of cholelithiasis during pregnancy, a cholecystectomy should be performed in the second trimester.

Similarly a pregnant woman with choledocholithiasis demonstrated on MRCP, ultrasound, or EUS should undergo therapeutic ERCP with minimization of radiation exposure.

TRIGLYCERIDE-INDUCED PANCREATITIS

Triglycerides increase 2- to 4-fold during pregnancy. This is attributed to the estrogen-mediated increase in hepatic production of triglyceride-rich lipoproteins in concert with the decrease in endothelial lipoprotein lipase activity.[2,5] In patients with an inborn error of lipoprotein metabolism, this can lead to triglyceride levels higher than 1000 mg/dL, which could precipitate pancreatitis. Though rare, accounting for only 4% to 6% of cases of pancreatitis during pregnancy, triglyceride-induced pancreatitis is often more severe and/or recurrent, poses management challenges, and is associated with a higher rate of preterm delivery.[5,9,16] Lipid lowering prior to conception, low-fat diet, intermittent lipid-free TPN, and fenofibrate have been recommended.[9,11] Omega-3 fatty acid supplementation may help to prevent pancreatitis.[16] Plasma exchange and heparin reportedly lead to a decrease in triglycerides, but the results are not sustained and, therefore, are not recommended.[8,9]

HYPERPARATHYROIDISM AND PANCREATITIS

Rarely, hyperparathyroidism is a cause of pancreatitis in nonpregnant patients occurring in 1% to 2% of patients. This increases during pregnancy to 7% to 13%.[3,17] Hyperparathyroidism can be managed conservatively with calcitonin and phosphates or surgically with parathyroidectomy performed ideally during the second trimester.

ALCOHOL

In one series, alcohol was found to contribute to 12% of cases.[5] However, in other studies, alcohol was not found to be a common cause of pancreatitis in pregnancy. It is widely accepted that alcohol is teratogenic, and alcohol consumption during pregnancy is not socially accepted.[18] This might lead patients to understate their use of alcohol during pregnancy. Pregnant patients who do use alcohol may present with acute or chronic pancreatitis during their pregnancy.

OUTCOMES IN PANCREATITIS

Historically, maternal mortality and perinatal mortality secondary to acute pancreatitis were high, with a 30% maternal death rate and a 60% fetal death rate.[19] Recent reports suggest dramatic improvement in survival. The rate of preterm delivery ranges from 20% to 40% and tends to be higher in patients who present during the first trimester or have more severe disease.[1,5,6,11] This rate is almost 3 times higher than the overall rate of preterm delivery, which is 12% in the United States according to the Centers for Disease Control. In biliary pancreatitis, preterm delivery is more common in those managed conservatively rather than surgically. The rate of fetal loss ranges from 3% to 11%,[1,5-7] but was as high as 33% in a retrospective review of pregnant patients with severe pancreatitis.[11] Maternal mortality is now rare. The severity of acute pancreatitis is related to maternal mortality. There were zero deaths in 4 series[1,5,7,11] and one death in one series, giving a mortality rate of 0.97%.[6] These improved outcomes are attributed to early recognition of pancreatitis and advances in medical and neonatal intensive care.

BILIARY DISEASE IN PREGNANCY

Pregnancy induces several physiologic changes in the gallbladder and biliary system, and there is an increased incidence of biliary disease during pregnancy. Changes in the gallbladder include an increase in the size/volume of the gallbladder, increased bile acid pool size, decreased enterohepatic circulation, decreased percentage of chenodeoxycholic acid, increased percentage of cholic acid, increased cholesterol secretion, and bile stasis.[2,8] This is likely mediated by progesterone and leads to the formation of supersaturated bile, cholesterol crystals, and subsequent gallstones.[2]

Biliary sludge is common and was found to develop in 31% of pregnant women followed from their first trimester through the immediate postpartum period.[20] Most of these women were asymptomatic, and sludge resolved by 5 months postpartum in two-thirds of the women. Gallstones were found to develop in 2% to 12% of pregnant women during the course of their pregnancy.[1,21] One-third of these patients developed symptoms, and one-third of these patients had resolution of gallstones postpartum.[16,17]

Despite the fact that gallstones are fairly common, complications of gallstones occur infrequently during pregnancy. The incidence of biliary colic was 0.09% and acute cholecystitis was 0.02% to 0.08%.[4,22] Choledocholithiasis and cholangitis are even rarer.[13] Acute pancreatitis was discussed in detail earlier.

BILIARY COLIC

Biliary colic, right upper quadrant pain in a patient with confirmed cholelithiasis, is more likely to occur in women with stones larger than 10 mm in diameter.[17] Initially, biliary colic should be managed with IV fluids and analgesics. For many patients, this is sufficient. However, the relapse rate of biliary colic is high and ranges from 40% to 60%.[4,10] Relapses occur more often when biliary colic presents in the first and second trimesters and result in more severe disease in 15% of cases, and may eventually require induction of labor due to refractory symptoms and preterm delivery.[4,10] Elective laparoscopic cholecystectomy performed during the late first or second trimesters is a reasonable option and is not associated with increased rates of preterm delivery or fetal loss.

ACUTE CHOLECYSTITIS

As in nonpregnant patients, acute cholecystitis in the pregnant patient presents with abdominal pain, vomiting, fever, anorexia, and leukocytosis.[2] There does not appear to be a correlation with gestational age. Medical management starts with IV fluids and analgesics. If there is concern for infection, antibiotics should be considered (see Table 10-1). In one series, medical management was "successful" 85% of the time; however, information regarding outcomes, such as rates of preterm delivery and fetal loss, was not provided.[18] A more recent analysis indicated that patients with acute cholecystitis are likely to fail medical management, and half required emergent surgery shortly after presentation.[4] Elective cholecystectomy is ideal for those who do not respond to medical management or who relapse and it can be safely performed during the second trimester of pregnancy.

GALLSTONE PANCREATITIS

See earlier section on pancreatitis.

CHOLEDOCHOLITHIASIS

Choledocholithiasis as a complication of biliary disease is rarely seen during pregnancy. It is diagnosed by the presence of gallstones in the common bile duct by ultrasound or MRCP. In addition to IV fluids, analgesics, and antibiotics for superimposed cholangitis,

ERCP with sphincterotomy is appropriate.[2] This may allow for postponement of cholecystectomy to the postpartum period. In studies describing 320 nonpregnant patients with gallstone pancreatitis or choledocholithiasis and gallbladder in situ managed by ERCP and sphincterotomy alone, three (1%) developed recurrent biliary pancreatitis, but 56 (17%) developed other biliary symptoms or complications (such as acute cholecystitis or biliary colic).[10]

KEY POINTS

- Biliary sludge develops in ~30% of pregnant women, and cholelithiasis develops in ~10% of pregnant women.
- Complications of cholelithiasis occur in <1% of pregnancies.
- ERCP can be performed safely in pregnancy.

REFERENCES

1. Ramin KD, Ramin SM, Richey SD, Cunningham FG. Acute pancreatitis in pregnancy. *Am J Obstet Gynecol.* 1995;173(1):187-191.
2. Ramin KD, Ramsey PS. Disease of the gallbladder and pancreas in pregnancy. *Obstet Gynecol Clin North Am.* 2001;28(3):571-580.
3. Stimac D, Stimac T. Acute pancreatitis during pregnancy. *Eur J Gastroenterol Hepatol.* 2011;doi:10.1097/MEG.0b013e328349b199.
4. Swisher SG, Schmit PJ, Hunt KK, et al. Biliary disease during pregnancy. *Am J Surg.* 1994;168(6):576-579; discussion 580-581.
5. Eddy JJ, Gideonsen MD, Song JY, Grobman WA, O'Halloran P. Pancreatitis in pregnancy. *Obstet Gynecol.* 2008;112(5):1075-1081.
6. Tang S-J, Rodriguez-Frias E, Singh S, et al. Acute pancreatitis during pregnancy. *Clin Gastroenterol Hepatol.* 2010;8(1):85-90.
7. Hernandez A, Petrov MS, Brooks DC, Banks PA, Ashley SW, Tavakkolizadeh A. Acute pancreatitis and pregnancy: A 10-year single center experience. *J Gastrointest Surg.* 2007;11(12):1623-1627.
8. Gupta K, Wu B. In the clinic. Acute pancreatitis. *Ann Intern Med.* 2010;153(9): ITC 51-55.
9. Talukdar R, Swaroop Vege S. Early management of severe acute pancreatitis. *Curr Gastroenterol Rep.* 2011;13(2):123-130.
10. Forsmark CE, Baillie J. AGA Institute Technical Review on acute pancreatitis. *Gastroenterology.* 2007;132:2022-2044.
11. Ranson JH, Pasternack BK. Statistical methods for quantifying the severity of clinical acute pancreatitis. *J Surg Res.* 1977;22(2):79-91.
12. Knaus WA, Draper EA, Wagner DP, Zimmerman JE. APACHE II: a severity of disease classification system. *Crit Care Med.* 1985;13(10):818-829.

13. Pitchumoni CS, Yegneswaran B. Acute pancreatitis in pregnancy. *World J Gastroenterol: WJG.* 2009;15(45):5641-5646.
14. Abu Musa AA, Usta IM, Rechdan JB, Nassar AH. Recurrent hypertriglyceridemia-induced pancreatitis in pregnancy: a management dilemma. *Pancreas.* 2006;32(2):227-228.
15. Lu EJ, Curet MJ, El-Sayed YY, Kirkwood KS. Medical versus surgical management of biliary tract disease in pregnancy. *Am J Surg.* 2004;188(6):755-759.
16. Takaishi K, Miyoshi J, Matsumura T, Honda R, Ohba T, Katabuchi H. Hypertriglyceridemic acute pancreatitis during pregnancy: prevention with diet therapy and omega-3 fatty acids in the following pregnancy. *Nutrition (Burbank, Los Angeles County, Calif.).* 2009;25(11-12):1094-1097.
17. Krysiak R, Wilk M, Okopien B. Recurrent pancreatitis induced by hyperparathyroidism in pregnancy. *Arch Gynecol Obstet.* 2011;284(3):531-534.
18. Papadakis E, Sarigianni M, Mikhailidis D, Mamopoulos A, Karagiannis V. Acute pancreatitis in pregnancy: an overview. *Eur J Obstet Gynecol ReprodBiol.* 2011;159(2):261-266.
19. Wilkinson E. Acute pancreatitis in pregnancy: a review of 98 cases and a report of 8 new cases. *Obstet Gynecol Surv.* 1973;28(5):281-303.
20. Maringhini A, Ciambra M, Baccelliere P, et al. Biliary sludge and gallstones in pregnancy: incidence, risk factors, and natural history. *Ann Intern Med.* 1993;119(2):116-120.
21. Valdivieso V, Covarrubias C, Siegel F, Cruz F. Pregnancy and cholelithiasis: pathogenesis and natural course of gallstones diagnosed in early puerperium. *Hepatology (Baltimore, Md.).* 1993;17(1):1-4.
22. Landers D, Carmona R, Crombleholme W, Lim R. Acute cholecystitis in pregnancy. *Obstet Gynecol.* 1987;69(1):131-133.

11

Chronic Liver Disease

Caitlyn M. Patrick, MD and
A. Sidney Barritt IV, MD, MSCR

Pregnancy in the setting of chronic liver disease is rare for several reasons. First, most women with advanced liver disease tend to be in their postreproductive years, with one study finding the prevalence of cirrhosis in reproductive-aged women to be approximately 45 cases per 100,000. Second, if the liver disease does progress earlier in these patients, they are typically infertile due to hormonal alterations caused by their liver disease that result in anovulation and amenorrhea.[1] Furthermore, there has historically been a high rate of maternal mortality in these patients as high as 10.5%.[2] However, given the advancements of medical therapies, this mortality rate has likely decreased, and there are increasing case reports of successful pregnancies in the literature. Therefore, it is important to understand how to manage these unique patients as therapy continues to improve.

There are several factors unique to patients with cirrhosis that predispose these patients and their fetuses to higher morbidity and mortality. These include the risk for spontaneous abortion, variceal bleeding, acute hepatic compensation, splenic artery aneurysm rupture, and postpartum hemorrhage.[3] Additionally, several of the

Isaacs KL, Long MD.
*GI and Liver Disease During Pregnancy:
A Practical Approach (pp. 167-184).*
© 2013 Taylor & Francis Group

medications typically used to treat the patient's disease process can have adverse effects on fetal growth and the ability to carry the pregnancy to term (Table 11-1). In this chapter, we will review the complications associated with cirrhosis and portal hypertension in the setting of the unique physiologic changes of pregnancy, and we will address recommendations for management. Safety data on medications used in chronic liver disease during pregnancy and breastfeeding are shown in Table 11-1. We will also discuss the therapies and complications relating to delivery in several chronic liver diseases, including chronic hepatitis B and C, autoimmune hepatitis, primary biliary cirrhosis, Wilson's disease, and nonalcoholic steatohepatitis (NASH), and then briefly review the treatment recommendations after liver transplant.

CIRRHOSIS AND PORTAL HYPERTENSION

The patient with cirrhosis should receive preconception counseling. As part of this counseling, the physician should discuss the increased risks associated with pregnancy, optimize medical therapy to prevent fetal harm, address the risk for passage of the predisposing viral or genetic disease to the patient's offspring, and make sure that pregnancy is delayed until the disease process is stabilized. If the patient is a candidate for liver transplant, then he or she should be advised to delay pregnancy until after transplantation due to improved outcomes. Additionally, the patient should be evaluated for esophageal varices, as the main risk factor associated with pregnancy is life-threatening bleeding secondary to variceal rupture with a mortality rate of 18% to 50%.

Esophageal variceal bleeding has been reported in 18% to 32% of pregnant women with cirrhosis and in up to 78% of those with known varices prior to pregnancy.[3] There are several factors that predispose these patients to an increased risk of rupture. In the last two trimesters of pregnancy, there is a significant increase in blood volume, and the growing uterus also places pressure on the inferior vena cava, causing this increased blood volume to be diverted through collaterals, which then leads to increased pressure within the esophageal veins. Furthermore, during labor, the increased abdominal pressure created via the Valsalva maneuver can lead to variceal bleeding.[4] In regard to prevention, prophylactic banding remains controversial with limited evidence of benefit,

Table 11-1

Medications Used for Chronic Liver Disease

Medication	FDA Pregnancy Category*	Pregnancy Comment	Breastfeeding Comment	Indication in Liver Disease
Propranolol	C	Adverse effects in animals. Beta blockers can cause intrauterine growth restriction (IUGR), small placentas, fetal/neonatal bradycardia, hypoglycemia, respiratory depression.	Probably safe, low levels secreted in breast milk	Prophylaxis for esophageal varices
Octreotide	B	No effects in animal studies	No studies but possibly safe, careful infant monitoring advised if used	Management of variceal bleeding
Furosemide	C	Reports of increased fetal urine production, electrolyte disturbances, and concern for decreased placental perfusion	No studies available, but theoretically diuresis may suppress lactation	Ascites
Spironolactone	C	Feminization of males in animal studies	Acceptable for use, negligible amount in breast milk	Ascites

(continued)

Table 11-1 (continued)

Medications Used for Chronic Liver Disease

Medication	FDA Pregnancy Category*	Pregnancy Comment	Breastfeeding Comment	Indication in Liver Disease
Lactulose	B	No effects in animal models	No studies available, unknown safety	Hepatic encephalopathy
Rifaximin	C	Adverse effects in high doses in animals, no human studies	No studies available, unknown safety	Hepatic encephalopathy
Lamivudine	C	Adverse effects in animal studies, no increased risk of birth defects reported in registries, increased risk of lactic acidosis in mothers	Probably unsafe. Adverse effects (neutropenia, severe anemia) noted in patients on this as part of HAART. No studies in HIV-negative mothers but the low doses for HBV therapy not expected to cause harm.	HBV treatment
Interferon-alpha	C	Caution due to antiproliferative activity, animal studies found abortifacient effect in high doses	Possibly safe, low levels secreted in breast milk with limited studies on effects in infants	HCV treatment
Ribavirin	X	Contraindicated, adverse effects in all animal studies	No studies available, unknown safety	HCV treatment

(continued)

Table 11-1 *(continued)*

Medications Used for Chronic Liver Disease

Medication	FDA Pregnancy Category*	Pregnancy Comment	Breastfeeding Comment	Indication in Liver Disease
Azathio-prine	D	Teratogenic in animals. IUGR, increased first trimester abortions, and congenital anomalies reported in humans	Possibly unsafe, no adverse effects in infants reported. If desired, consider avoiding breastfeeding for 4 to 6 hours after a dose.	Autoimmune hepatitis
Cortico-steroids	C (D in 1st trimester)	Adverse effects in animal studies, association with oral cleft defects reported in first trimester	Probably safe, limited studies	Autoimmune hepatitis
Ursodeoxy-cholic acid	B	No effects in animal studies	Probably safe, limited studies	PBC
Hydro-xyzine	C	Adverse effects at high doses in animal studies, risk for neonatal withdrawal syndrome	No studies available, unknown safety	PBC
D-Penicil-lamine	D	Birth defects reported but should continue use for Wilson's disease with dose <500 mg/day and <250 mg in last 6 weeks of gestation	Probably unsafe, enters breast milk with limited studies on infant effects	Wilson's disease

(continued)

Table 11-1 (continued)

Medications Used for Chronic Liver Disease

Medication	FDA Pregnancy Category*	Pregnancy Comment	Breastfeeding Comment	Indication in Liver Disease
Trientine	C	Adverse effects in animal studies	No studies available, unknown safety	Wilson's disease
Zinc sulfate	C	Sufficient data not available	No studies available, unknown safety	Wilson's disease
Tacrolimus	C	Adverse effects in animal studies, neonatal hyperkalemia and renal dysfunction reported	Possibly safe, low amount secreted in breast milk, no adverse effects reported in infants	Transplant recipients
Cyclosporine	C	No adverse effects in animal studies, reports of premature birth and low birth weight in humans	Possibly unsafe, variable amounts enter breast milk	Transplant recipients
Mycophenolate	D	Adverse effects in animal studies, associated with congenital malformations and spontaneous abortions	No studies available, unknown safety	Transplant recipients

Adapted from Tan J, Surti B, Saab S. Pregnancy and cirrhosis. *Liver Transpl*. 2008;14(8):1081-1091; Wakim-Fleming J, Zein NN. Liver diseases in pregnancy. *Pregnancy in Gastrointestinal Disorders. American College of Gastroenterology Monographs*; updated 2007. https://www.acg.gi.org; Lexicomp Online. Lexi-Comp Inc; 2011. http://online.lexi.com. Accessed October 2011; and LactMed. National Library of Medicine; 2011. http://toxnet.nlm.nih.gov/cgi-bin/sis/htmlgen?LACT. Accessed October 2011.

*See Appendix for discussion of FDA pregnancy categories.

but in women at high risk for bleeding, the benefits of treatment with a nonselective beta blocker, such as propranolol (Pregnancy Category C), may outweigh the risks of potential fetal harm and should be discussed with the patient.[5] The best method of delivery also remains controversial because of the increased risk of rupture associated with the straining during the second stage of labor. Early epidural anesthesia is preferred, and most experts tend to recommend forceps or vacuum-assisted delivery. Elective C-section can also be performed, but there is an increased risk of bleeding from pelvic or abdominal collaterals.[4,6]

If variceal bleeding does occur, then the patient should be managed acutely with blood products and endoscopic intervention in the same manner as the noncirrhotic patient. However, while the use of octreotide is considered safe (Category B) in pregnant patients, vasopressin is contraindicated because it has been shown to be teratogenic.[1] If variceal bleeding is unable to be controlled endoscopically, then rescue therapy with placement of a transhepatic portosystemic shunt (TIPS) can be considered as a last resort, but there are only 3 cases of TIPS placement reported in the literature and the procedure is generally contraindicated due to the risk of radiation exposure to the fetus.[3]

Additional risks during pregnancy in cirrhotic patents include hepatic decompensation, hepatic encephalopathy, splenic artery aneurysm rupture, and postpartum uterine hemorrhage. Hepatic decompensation can occur during any stage of pregnancy and can be seen in up to 24% of patients, usually following an episode of variceal bleeding.[6] In cases of fulminant hepatic failure, a limited number of successful liver transplants have been reported; however, these tend to be in patients without pre-existing cirrhosis.[1] Ascites is rare in pregnancy given the increased intra-abdominal pressure but, if necessary, patients can be managed with diuretics, with both furosemide and spironolactone classified as Category C.[3] Hepatic encephalopathy occurs due to the same precipitating factors as in nonpregnant cirrhotics and can be managed with lactulose (Category B) and treatment of the precipitating factors. Pregnant patients are at a particularly higher risk of splenic aneurysm rupture: 20% of cases occur during pregnancy with 70% being in the third trimester. These patients tend to have few warning symptoms, including left upper quadrant pain, nausea, and syncope before developing acute hemorrhagic shock.[7] They should be treated with emergency splenectomy, transcatheter embolization, or stent-graft placement.[8] Finally, cirrhotic patients are at an increased risk of postpartum hemorrhage likely due to the increased incidence of coagulopathy and thrombocytopenia in these patients. These patients should be managed in the same manner as noncirrhotic patients with transfusion of blood products, use of oxytocin, and surgical intervention if necessary.[3]

KEY POINTS
• Pregnancy in cirrhotic patients is rare, but not contraindicated with the appropriate monitoring.   • Preconception counseling should occur with all patients of reproductive age with cirrhosis to ensure the best outcome.   • Maternal and fetal mortality is higher in patients with cirrhosis. The main risks are associated with variceal bleeding.

CHRONIC HEPATITIS B

Pregnant patients are routinely tested for hepatitis B virus (HBV) mainly because of the risks associated with perinatal transmission. Generally, patients with chronic HBV do not have any issues with fertility and do well during pregnancy if their disease has not progressed to cirrhosis.[9] All markers of liver function decrease during pregnancy because of the increased extracellular volume with the exception of alkaline phosphatase, which is produced by the placenta. However, later in pregnancy, the ALT level and hepatitis B viral load tend to increase significantly with studies showing a 0.4-log increase in viral load, particularly in HBeAg-positive patients.[10] The biggest risk for vertical transmission of infection is the maternal viral level. In endemic areas, the neonate has an 80% to 90% risk of becoming a chronic carrier if the mother is a chronic HBsAg carrier with a detectable viral level,[11] but this rate is decreased to 10% to 30% if the viral level is undetectable.[9] Antiviral treatment during pregnancy remains controversial as there are no long-term studies on outcomes available, but a recent small trial by Kose and colleagues has shown that, in patients with high viral levels, it can be effective and safe to prevent transmission with lamivudine treatment (Category C) during the last month of pregnancy.[12] C-section is not currently recommended because studies have not shown a significant decrease in transmission of infection.[13] To prevent transmission, all infants born to HBsAg-positive mothers should receive the hepatitis B vaccine series as well as the hepatitis B immunoglobulin within 12 hours of giving birth. Breastfeeding is generally encouraged after the hepatitis B immunoglobulin has been given; however, there have been some studies that indicate that HBV can be transmitted via breast milk and that the mother should be instructed to take good care of her nipples to prevent cracking and bleeding, which can increase the risk of transmission.[9]

KEY POINTS
• Chronic HBV infection does not increase morbidity and mortality in the setting of stable liver disease. • The main risk associated with chronic infection is vertical transmission to the neonate, which can be prevented with both the vaccine series and the administration of hepatitis B immunoglobulin. • Antiviral treatment during pregnancy has not been well-studied but may be effective in the last month of pregnancy.

CHRONIC HEPATITIS C

In contrast to chronic HBV infection, chronic hepatitis C virus (HCV) is associated with a lower risk of vertical transmission with rates between 4% and 10%; therefore, it is typically only recommended to perform HCV antibody screening in women with risk factors for infection, including a history of intravenous drug use or prior blood transfusions as well as tattoos or body piercings.[9] Patients with chronic HCV infection do not have an increased risk of adverse outcomes if their liver disease is well-controlled. As with HBV infection, the main risk for vertical transmission occurs in patients with higher viral levels during their pregnancy.[14] Additionally, patients with HIV co-infection are at an increased risk for perinatal transmission, which is thought to be due to impaired immune function leading to a higher rate of HCV viral replication. In these patients, antiretroviral treatment for HIV decreases the rate of HCV transmission to that of non-HIV-infected patients.[15] Conversely, antiviral treatment for HCV is not currently recommended, even in patients with high viral levels due to the high risk of birth defects associated with ribavirin, which is classified as Category X. Additionally, while interferon does not appear to have an adverse effect on the fetus, it has known antiproliferative activity, and there are limited studies of its effects so it should also be avoided during pregnancy (Category C).[9]

There are conflicting data about the risk of transmission associated with a vaginal birth. A recent multicenter European trial did not demonstrate a reduced rate of transmission with C-section[16]; however, older studies have demonstrated a significantly increased rate of transmission in vaginally delivered infants.[17] It should also be noted that, despite the mode of delivery, there is an increased risk of transmission with prolonged rupture of the membranes and invasive fetal monitoring.[3] There are currently no vaccines or immunoglobulins available for HCV, and it should be noted that, due to the transmission of maternal antibodies to the fetus through the placenta, the early presence of antibodies does not indicate infection. If the infant has the presence of HCV RNA at 3 to 6 months of age or persistence of HCV antibodies after 18 months, then he or she is considered infected.[14] Breastfeeding is generally considered safe, with several studies demonstrating no increased risk of transmission, so all major health agencies recommend breastfeeding.[9] On the other hand, it is possible to detect HCV RNA in breast milk, particularly in patients with very high viral levels, so some authors recommend against breastfeeding in these select patients.[18]

KEY POINTS

- Screening for HCV is only indicated in patients with risk factors.
- Treatment for HCV should be delayed until after pregnancy due to the teratogenic effects of ribavirin.
- There is conflicting evidence about the preferred mode of delivery, but more recent data suggest there is no increased benefit with C-section.

AUTOIMMUNE HEPATITIS

Autoimmune hepatitis typically affects young women and can cause infertility, with oligomenorrhea being a presenting symptom. However, with immunosuppressive treatment and control of the disease, normal menstrual cycles can recur and successful pregnancy can be achieved.[19] Maternal and fetal complications tend to be higher in these patients, with a fetal loss rate reported as high as 24%.[20] Disease activity in these patients is variable, with some patients experiencing an improvement in their disease possibly secondary to the immune tolerance induced by pregnancy, whereas others can experience a disease flare. Because of the risks associated with a disease flare during pregnancy, it is recommended to continue treatment throughout the pregnancy. Azathioprine (Category D) can be used to maintain remission, and it has been used in pregnant women with inflammatory bowel disease with good results at doses less than 100 mg/day.[21] Corticosteroids (Category C) can be used to induce remission if a flare should occur and can also be used in higher doses if azathioprine withdrawal is desired during the pregnancy.[19] Additionally, some studies recommend decreasing azathioprine doses after the third month of pregnancy, as liver tests typically improve during this period of time. However, it is usually necessary to increase the amount of immunosuppression in the postpartum period when the risk for a disease flare is highest.[3] Breastfeeding on azathioprine is considered "probably safe" as it is minimally excreted in the milk, and a recent study did not show any adverse effects in breastfed infants.[19]

KEY POINTS
• Pregnancy can be achieved in patients with good disease control.
• Treatment should be continued throughout pregnancy to prevent flares.

PRIMARY BILIARY CIRRHOSIS

Primary biliary cirrhosis (PBC) is a rare condition with 90% of affected patients being women 35 to 60 years of age. These patients are typically infertile with only rare case reports of pregnant patients with this disease in the literature. Most of these cases noted deterioration of liver function during pregnancy. Those cases that progressed to the third trimester were complicated by jaundice, which could be caused by increased estrogen levels leading to cholestasis.[22] Treatment with ursodeoxycholic acid (Category B) has been shown to be safe and effective to help treat pruritus in patients with PBC in one study,[23] but some authorities suggest that it should not be used in the first trimester. Hydroxyzine (Category C) is contraindicated in early pregnancy.[3] Additionally, PBC leads to malabsorption of vitamins A, D, and K and calcium, so these should be supplemented during pregnancy.[22]

KEY POINTS
• Pregnancy in patients with PBC is rare. • Urodeoxycholic acid can be used for treatment.

WILSON'S DISEASE

Wilson's disease is a rare autosomal recessive disease affecting copper transport, which leads to copper accumulation in several organs including the liver and brain. Symptoms typically develop in the teenage years to early 20s, affecting women of reproductive age. Prior to treatment, these patients may have irregular menses with multiple miscarriages, because excess copper can interfere with ovarian follicular aromatase activity in addition to the effects that liver disease itself has on fertility.[24] In patients who become pregnant, it is important to continue treatment because discontinuation can lead to disease regression, fulminant liver failure, and possibly death.[25] There are 3 anti-copper agents that can be used to treat Wilson's disease, including D-penicillamine (Category D), trientine (Category C), and zinc (Category C). If D-penicillamine or trientine are used, there should be a 25% to 50% reduction in prepregnancy doses to prevent copper depletion and poor wound healing in the event of a C-section. D-penicillamine has also been associated with a teratogenic syndrome called cutis laxa syndrome; however, these effects are typically seen at higher doses, so it is suggested to decrease the dose to less than 500 mg/day during pregnancy.[21] Zinc therapy has a different mechanism of action than the chelating agents and does not need to be dose-adjusted during pregnancy.[25] It is also considered safe to use during breastfeeding, unlike D-penicillamine and trientene.[21]

KEY POINT
• Therapy needs to be continued throughout pregnancy to prevent disease regression.

NONALCOHOLIC STEATOHEPATITIS

There are limited studies on the effects of nonalcoholic steatohepatitis during pregnancy but as the disease becomes more prevalent in our population, guidelines for treatment during pregnancy should be further clarified. A recent study suggests that the diagnosis of nonalcoholic fatty liver disease should be considered when other causes for abnormal liver enzyme elevations in pregnancy are ruled out. This patient population with signs of the metabolic syndrome is at an increased risk of disease progression following pregnancy, and recognizing these liver enzyme abnormalities early is helpful for prevention. These patients should be educated on the lifestyle modifications they can adopt to prevent progression of their liver disease. They should also be screened for gestational diabetes and counseled against gaining excessive weight during their pregnancy.[26]

KEY POINT
• Pregnant patients with the metabolic syndrome and unexplained elevation of liver enzymes should be educated on lifestyle modifications.

PREGNANCY AFTER LIVER TRANSPLANT

As discussed above, cirrhosis and end-stage liver disease usually lead to infertility; however, after liver transplant, 80% of premenopausal women will have a return of normal menstrual cycles within 1 year.[14] These patients should be instructed to continue contraception use for at least 1 year after transplant, as this results in a higher rate of successful live births and lower rates of graft rejection. This is because in the early post-transplant period patients require higher levels of immunosuppression and are at increased risk of graft rejection. They are also more susceptible to infection, including acute cytomegalovirus infection, which can be detrimental to the developing fetus.[27] Immunosuppressive therapy should be continued throughout the pregnancy. All currently used medications including tacrolimus, cyclosporine, mycophenolate, sirolimus, and prednisone are classified as Category C drugs because their effects on the fetus have not been well-studied.[14] Studies have shown that these patients are at an increased risk of pregnancy-induced hypertension and pre-eclampsia, which may be related to their immunosuppressive medications.[28] These patients also tend to have an increased rate of premature births and low birth weight babies compared to the general population. The rate of graft rejection does not appear to be affected by pregnancy with acute rejection rates similar to their nonpregnant counterparts.[29]

KEY POINTS

- Most patients regain fertility after transplant, but should be advised to use contraception for at least 1 year after transplant.
- Immunosuppressive medications should be continued throughout pregnancy.

SUMMARY

While pregnancy in the setting of chronic liver disease is rare, improvements in therapy will likely increase the incidence of successful pregnancies. Therefore, physicians should be aware of the unique implications the disease process has on the mother and fetus, as well as the appropriate medications that are safe for use during pregnancy. Patients with cirrhosis and portal hypertension have a significant increase in maternal complications and need to be closely monitored. Chronic viral hepatitis does not tend to adversely affect pregnancy if the patient has not yet developed cirrhosis but does increase the risk for transmission of infection to the fetus. This requires special considerations for treatment during pregnancy and at delivery. Pregnancy in patients with chronic diseases including autoimmune hepatitis, PBC, and Wilson's disease is rare with small studies available for treatment recommendations. The main recommendations of these studies involve continuing treatment throughout the pregnancy with appropriate modifications in the medication regimen as noted previously. Finally, special consideration should be given to post liver transplant recipients, as they are very likely to regain fertility and should be counseled on the appropriate contraception and timing of pregnancy, as well as the risks associated with becoming pregnant while remaining on immunosuppressive medication.

REFERENCES

1. Russell MA, Craigo SD. Cirrhosis and portal hypertension in pregnancy. *Semin Perinatol.* 1998;22(12):156-165.
2. Steven MM. Pregnancy and liver disease. *Gut.* 1981;22(7):592-614.
3. Tan J, Surti B, Saab S. Pregnancy and cirrhosis. *Liver Transpl.* 2008;14(8): 1081-1091.
4. Rosenfeld H, Hochner-Celniker D, Ackerman Z. Massive bleeding from ectopic varices in the postpartum period: rare but serious complication in women with portal hypertension. *Eur J Gastroenterol Hepatol.* 2009;21(9):1086-1091.
5. Garcia-Tsao G, Sanyal AJ, Grace ND, Carey W. Practice Guidelines Committee of the American Association for the study of liver diseases, and practice parameters committee of the American College of Gastroenterology. Prevention and management of gastroesophageal varices and variceal hemorrhage in cirrhosis. *Hepatology.* 2007;46:922-938.
6. Benjaminov FS, Heathcote J. Liver disease in pregnancy. *Am J Gastroenterol.* 2004;99(12):2479-2488.
7. O'Grady JP, Day EJ, Toole AL, Paust JC. Splenic artery aneurysm in pregnancy. *Obstet Gynecol.* 1977;50(5):627-630.
8. Pasha SF, Glovicki P, Stanson AW, Kamath PS. Splanchnic artery aneurysms. *Mayo Clin Proc.* 2007;82(4):472-479.
9. Sookoian S. Effect of pregnancy on pre-existing liver disease: chronic viral hepatitis. *Ann Hepatol.* 2006;5(3):190-197.

10. Soderstrom A, Norkrans G, Lindh M. Hepatitis B virus DNA during pregnancy and post partum: aspects of vertical transmission. *Scand J Infect Dis.* 1994;170(6):1418-1423.

11. Lee C, Gong Y, Brok J, Boxall EH, Gluud C. Effect of hepatitis B immunization in newborn infants of mothers positive for hepatitis B surface antigen: systematic review and meta-analysis. *BMJ.* 2006;11;332(7537):328-336.

12. Köse S, Türken M, Devrim I, Taner C. Efficacy and safety of lamivudine treatment in late pregnancy with high HBV DNA: a perspective for mother and infants. *J Infect Dev Ctries.* 2011;26;5(4):303-306.

13. Wang J, Zhu Q, Zhang X. Effect of delivery mode on maternal-infant transmission of hepatitis B virus by immunoprophylaxis. *Clin Med J (Engl).* 2002;115(10):1510-1512.

14. Martin A, Sass D. Liver disease in pregnancy. *Gastroenterol Clin North Am.* 2011;40(2):335-353, viii.

15. Conte D, Fraquelli M, Prati D, Colucci A, Minola E. Prevalence and clinical course of chronic hepatitis C virus (HCV) infection and rate of HCV vertical transmission in a cohort of 15,250 pregnant women. *Hepatology.* 2000;31(3):751-755.

16. European Pediatric Hepatitis C Virus Network. A significant sex—but not elective cesarean section—effect on mother-to-child transmission of hepatitis C virus infection. *J Infect Dis.* 2005;192(11):1872-1879.

17. Paccagnini S, Principi N, Massironi E, et al. Perinatal transmission and manifestation of hepatitis C virus infection in a high risk population. *Pediatr Infect Dis J.* 1995;14(3):195-199.

18. Kumar RM, Shahul S. Role of breast-feeding in transmission of hepatitis C virus to infants of HCV-infected mothers. *J Hepatol.* 1998;29(2):191-197.

19. Aggarwal N, Chopra S, Suri V, Sikka P, Dhiman R, Chawla Y. Pregnancy outcome in women with autoimmune hepatitis. *Arch Gynecol Obstet.* 2011;284(1):19-23.

20. Schramm C, Herkel J, Beuers U, Kanzler S, Galle PR, Lohse AW. Pregnancy in autoimmune hepatitis. Outcome and risk factors. *Am J Gastroenterol.* 2006;101(3):556-560.

21. Wakim-Fleming J, Zein NN. Liver diseases in pregnancy. *Pregnancy in Gastrointestinal Disorders. American College of Gastroenterology Monographs*; updated 2007. https://www.acg.gi.org.

22. Goh SK, Gull SE, Alexander GJ. Pregnancy in primary biliary cirrhosis complicated by portal hypertension: report of a case and review of the literature. *BJOG.* 2001;108(7):760-762.

23. Rudi J, Schonig T, Stremmel W. Therapy with ursodeoxycholic acid in primary biliary cirrhosis in pregnancy. *Z Gastroenterol.* 1996;34(3):188-191.

24. Kaushanksy A, Frydman M, Kaufman H, Homburg R. Endocrine studies of the ovulatory disturbances in Wilson's disease. *Fertil Steril.* 1987;47(2):270-273.

25. Brewer GJ, Johnson VD, Dick RD, Hedera P, Fink JK, Kluin KJ. Treatment of Wilson's disease with zinc. XVII: treatment during pregnancy. *Hepatology.* 2000;31(2):364-370.

26. Page LM, Girling JC. A novel cause for abnormal liver function tests in pregnancy and the puerperium: nonalcoholic fatty liver disease. *BJOG.* 2011;118(12):1532-1535.

27. Christopher V, Al-Chalabi T, Richardson PD, et al. Pregnancy outcome after liver transplantation: a single-center experience of 71 pregnancies in 45 recipients. *Liver Transpl.* 2006;12(7):1138-1143.

28. Nagy S, Bush MC, Berkowitz R, Fishbein TM, Gomez-Lobo V. Pregnancy outcome in liver transplant recipients. *Obstet Gynecol.* 2003;102(1):121-128.

29. Armenti VT, Radomski JS, Moritz MJ, et al. Report from the National Transplant Pregnancy Registry (NTPR): outcomes of pregnancy after transplantation. *Clin Transpl.* 2005:69-83.

30. Lexicomp Online. Lexi-Comp Inc; 2011. http://online.lexi.com. Accessed October 2011.

31. LactMed. National Library of Medicine; 2011. http://toxnet.nlm.nih.gov/cgi-bin/sis/htmlgen?LACT. Accessed October 2011.

12

Acute Liver Disease

Eric S. Orman, MD and
A. Sidney Barritt IV, MD, MSCR

Acute liver injury (ALI) occurs uncommonly during pregnancy, with an estimated incidence of 3%.[1] Despite its rarity, awareness of acute liver dysfunction is important due to its associated morbidity and mortality. Furthermore, prompt recognition and identification of a specific etiology is important because early and specific intervention may improve patient outcomes (eg, anticoagulation for Budd-Chiari syndrome or early delivery for acute fatty liver of pregnancy). Acute liver disease can be categorized into 2 groups: general liver diseases that occur coincidentally during a pregnancy, and those that are unique to the pregnant patient (Table 12-1). In this chapter, we will review both of these groups with an emphasis on those diseases unique to the pregnant patient.

THE LIVER IN NORMAL PREGNANCY

When evaluating a patient for suspected acute liver disease, it is important to recall the variations in liver-related findings and tests that result from normal maternal physiologic and hormonal changes.

185

Isaacs KL, Long MD.
GI and Liver Disease During Pregnancy:
A Practical Approach (pp. 185-210).
© 2013 Taylor & Francis Group

Table 12-1

Characteristics of Liver Diseases

Condition	Trimester	Clinical Findings	AST, ALT	Bilirubin	Diagnosis	Treatment
Not Unique to Pregnancy						
Acute hepatitis A	Any	Nausea, vomiting, anorexia, abdominal pain, jaundice	+++	++	Anti-HAV IgM	Supportive
Acute hepatitis B	Any	Nausea, vomiting, anorexia, abdominal pain, jaundice	+++	+/-	HBsAg, anti-HBc IgM, HBeAg, HBV DNA	Supportive, antiviral therapy rarely needed
Acute hepatitis E	Any	Nausea, vomiting, anorexia, abdominal pain, jaundice	+++	++	Anti-HEV, HEV RNA (research labs only)	Supportive
Budd-Chiari syndrome	Any	Abdominal pain, ascites	++	+	Doppler ultrasound, MRI	Anticoagulation
DILI	Any	Variable	++	+/-	History	Stop drug +/- N-acetylcysteine

(continued)

Table 12-1 *(continued)*

Characteristics of Liver Diseases

Condition	Trimester	Clinical Findings	AST, ALT	Bilirubin	Diagnosis	Treatment
Unique to Pregnancy						
HG	1	Nausea, vomiting, dehydration	++	-	History	Thiamine, antiemetics, nutrition
ICP	2, 3	Pruritus	++	+	History, elevated serum bile acids	UDCA
Pre-eclampsia, HELLP	2, 3, post	Hypertension, headache, abdominal pain, edema, seizures	++	-	Hypertension, proteinuria, hemolysis, thrombocytopenia	Delivery
AFLP	3	Nausea, vomiting, abdominal pain	++	+	History, labs, imaging	Delivery

DILI: drug-induced liver injury; HG: hyperemesis gravidarum; ICP: intrahepatic cholestasis of pregnancy; HELLP: hemolysis, elevated liver enzymes, low platelets; AFLP: acute fatty liver of pregnancy

Spider angiomas and palmar erythema can be present due to hyperestrogenemia.[2] Because of hemodilution, serum albumin levels are decreased in all trimesters, and mild thrombocytopenia is common.[3] Serum alkaline phosphatase increases late in pregnancy owing to production of a placental isoenzyme.[4] Other liver biochemical tests may change slightly but remain within normal limits.[5] Grossly and microscopically, the liver is unchanged during pregnancy.

KEY POINTS

- Serum albumin is decreased in pregnancy.
- Alkaline phosphatase is increased in the last trimester.

SYMPTOMS AND SIGNS

The clinical presentation of the pregnant woman with ALI is similar to that of the nonpregnant patient. Symptoms are typically nonspecific and may include abdominal pain, nausea, vomiting, jaundice, and pruritus, although patients can be asymptomatic. The development of hepatic encephalopathy is an ominous sign and should prompt urgent evaluation and referral to a hepatologist. ALI can occur at any point during pregnancy, but the timing and symptoms can often be clues to the specific etiology (eg, hyperemesis gravidarum in the first-trimester patient with nausea and vomiting). A detailed medical history is essential. In particular, the patient should be questioned regarding complications or liver-related symptoms during prior pregnancies; any previous history of liver disease or abnormal liver biochemical tests; risk factors for liver diseases including injection drug use, travel, and high-risk behaviors; and a detailed medication history. For patients with suggestive signs or symptoms, a systematic evaluation should be performed to diagnose ALI, establish an etiology, and exclude extrahepatic disease. This should include general liver biochemical testing including the prothrombin time and an ultrasound examination of the liver in addition to more specific testing, if appropriate.

KEY POINTS
• Timing of onset and symptoms are crucial in making a correct diagnosis.
• Laboratory evaluation should be based on the history.
• Liver biopsy is rarely needed.

DISEASES NOT UNIQUE TO PREGNANCY

ACUTE HEPATITIS A

The hepatitis A virus (HAV) is transmitted by the fecal-oral route and causes an acute hepatitis that is usually self-limited, only rarely resulting in a fulminant course.[6] The incidence of infection in Western nations is low and has only rarely been reported in pregnant patients.[7] Often, patients present with jaundice, and typically the aminotransferases are greater than 1000 IU/L. The diagnosis is established by the presence of serum anti-HAV IgM antibodies; after recovery from infection, anti-HAV IgG antibodies will persist long-term and provide natural immunity to re-infection. HAV infection in the second and third trimesters has been associated with an increase in the risk of gestational complications leading to preterm labor, but neonatal outcomes are generally favorable.[8] Fever and hypoalbuminemia may predict preterm labor. Only a few cases of vertical transmission of HAV have been reported, with generally good neonatal outcomes.[7] Pregnant women at risk for HAV should be vaccinated, and those with a potential exposure should also receive immune globulin.[9] Treatment is supportive, as the disease is typically self-limited.

KEY POINTS
• At-risk women should be vaccinated for HAV.
• Anti-HAV IgM is required to diagnose acute HAV.
• Treatment of acute HAV is supportive.

ACUTE HEPATITIS B

In the Western world, hepatitis B is typically transmitted via sexual contact or blood exposure, and acute infection is clinically apparent in a minority of patients. Of adults with acute HBV, less than 1% has a fulminant course, and only a small minority progress to chronic infection.[10] Following an incubation period of 4 to 20 weeks, patients can present with nonspecific symptoms such as nausea, abdominal discomfort, and jaundice. Symptom onset may occur during the late first or early second trimester if the infection is acquired at the time of conception. Like HAV, the aminotransferases can rise up to 2000 IU/L, with the ALT typically greater than the AST. Acute infection is diagnosed by the presence of surface antigen (HBsAg) and anticore (HBc) IgM antibody in the serum. Hepatitis B e antigen (HBeAg) and HBV DNA can also be detected. Distinguishing acute infection from an exacerbation of chronic infection can be challenging, as these laboratory markers can be seen in both conditions. Knowledge of the epidemiology and natural history of hepatitis B is important in making this distinction. Like HAV, preterm birth may be more common in the setting of acute HBV, but rates of spontaneous abortion, stillbirth, and congenital malformations are not increased.[11] However, more than half of women with acute infection near delivery will transmit the virus to the neonate with a very high risk of resultant chronic infection.[12] Accordingly, pregnant women at risk for acute infection should be vaccinated,[13] and those with possible exposure to HBV should also receive hepatitis B immune globulin. Treatment for acute HBV is primarily supportive. In general, only a minority of patients (ie, those with fulminant disease or with protracted, severe disease) requires specific antiviral therapy.[14] Direct antiviral therapy for acute HBV has not been studied in the context of pregnancy. Therapy for chronic HBV will be discussed in Chapter 11.

KEY POINTS

- At-risk women should be vaccinated for HBV.
- HBsAg, anti-HBc IgM, and HBV DNA should be obtained if suspicious for acute HBV.
- Treatment is usually supportive; specific antiviral therapy may be considered in consultation with a hepatologist.

ACUTE HEPATITIS E

Hepatitis E virus (HEV) is an enterally transmitted pathogen that is endemic in the developing world. A detailed travel history should be obtained when considering this diagnosis; almost all cases of acute infection in Western countries have occurred in patients with recent travel to endemic areas. However, pockets of endemic areas and high-risk professions are being discovered within the United States, particularly within the pig farming industry.[15] Clinically, its effects are similar to the other viral hepatitides. The diagnosis can be challenging as no tests for HEV have been approved for commercial use in the United States, although tests for anti-HEV antibodies and ribonucleic acid (RNA) PCR can be performed by research laboratories. Although HEV typically follows a self-limited course, multiple studies have highlighted the increased incidence and severity of illness in the setting of pregnancy. In one series, 17.3% of pregnant women developed acute hepatitis compared to nonpregnant women (2.1%) and men (2.8%) during an epidemic of HEV.[16] In another large prospective study, HEV-infected pregnant patients were more likely to have obstetric complications and poor fetal outcomes compared with non-HEV acute viral hepatitis. In addition, more than half of the infected pregnant patients developed acute liver failure, with an overall mortality rate of 41%.[17] The reasons for the severe outcomes seen in the pregnant patient are not clear, but may be related to increased viral replication.[18] Vertical transmission has been reported as well and is associated with poor neonatal outcomes.[19] Current treatment for acute HEV infection is supportive; there are no specific antiviral therapies for this infection. Although vaccines are in development,[20] none are currently available for clinical use. To prevent infection, travelers to endemic areas should avoid drinking unpurified water and eating uncooked fruits and vegetables.

KEY POINTS
• Acute HEV may be more common and more severe in pregnant women.
• Diagnostic tests are not FDA approved but are available in research laboratories.
• Treatment of acute HEV is supportive.

BUDD-CHIARI SYNDROME

Budd-Chiari syndrome refers to hepatic venous outflow obstruction, most commonly manifest as thrombosis of the hepatic veins or inferior vena cava. This obstruction results in venous stasis and congestion, leading to hepatocyte necrosis and fibrosis. The clinical presentation depends on the rapidity of the venous occlusion, and patients can be classified as fulminant, acute, subacute, or chronic. Only a minority of patients present with solely "acute" symptoms, most often ascites and abdominal pain.[21] In the fulminant and acute forms, transaminases can be several hundred IU/L, with higher values indicative of more severe disease.[22] The diagnosis requires a radiologic study to demonstrate vascular occlusion. Typically, this can be achieved with Doppler ultrasound, contrast-enhanced CT, or MRI. If these studies are not diagnostic but clinical suspicion is high, the gold standard test is direct venography of the hepatic veins. Tests using ionizing radiation should be performed judiciously in the pregnant patient with appropriate precautions for the fetus. Budd-Chiari syndrome is rare and most patients have at least one thrombotic risk factor, most commonly a myeloproliferative disorder.[21] Oral contraceptive use and pregnancy are associated with an increased risk of hepatic vein thrombosis, but usually in the setting of another underlying thrombotic risk factor.[23] Thus, a comprehensive evaluation for additional thrombotic risk factors should be undertaken. Treatment should be coordinated with a liver transplant center. Although therapy has not been systematically evaluated in pregnant patients, in general, initial therapy consists of anticoagulation with heparin (avoiding vitamin K antagonists in the pregnant patient) and angioplasty of amenable vascular lesions, followed by transjugular intrahepatic portosystemic shunt placement for those without improvement and consideration of liver transplantation.[24] Despite a historically high mortality, with contemporary therapies, prognosis has improved with a 5-year transplant-free survival rate of 78%.[25] Nevertheless, poor fetal outcomes have been described.[23]

> **KEY POINTS**
>
> - Pregnant women with acute Budd-Chiari syndrome should be evaluated for other thrombotic risk factors.
> - Diagnosis of Budd-Chiari requires Doppler ultrasound or contrast-enhanced MRI.
> - Treatment should be coordinated with a liver transplant center.

AUTOIMMUNE HEPATITIS

Although classified as a chronic disease, autoimmune hepatitis (AIH) can rarely present in an acute severe or fulminant form. However, the immune-tolerant state induced by pregnancy often results in quiescence of AIH, and acute AIH during pregnancy is extremely rare.[26] This disease entity, which is primarily treated with corticosteroids, should nevertheless be entertained when evaluating the pregnant patient with ALI. The diagnosis is clinical and is based on the presence of serum autoimmune serologies and typical histologic findings. The management of patients who become pregnant with a known diagnosis of AIH was discussed in Chapter 11.

> **KEY POINT**
>
> - Acute autoimmune hepatitis is extremely rare in pregnancy.

DRUG-INDUCED LIVER INJURY

Drug-induced liver injury (DILI) is the most common cause of acute liver failure in the United States[27] and is the most common reason that new medications fail to achieve FDA approval.[28] Clinically, DILI has a highly variable presentation, and patterns of biochemical test abnormalities can range from hepatocellular (with predominant aminotransferase elevations) to cholestatic (with elevations in the bilirubin and alkaline phosphatase). DILI carries a significant mortality rate, particularly in those with a hepatocellular pattern of injury and concurrent jaundice.[29] DILI has rarely been reported in pregnant patients and most reports have been associated with antiretroviral therapy,[30] commonly used to prevent vertical transmission of HIV, and alpha-methyldopa,[31] an antihypertensive commonly used in pregnancy. Fatal outcomes during pregnancy have been reported.[32] The primary treatment of DILI is withdrawal of the offending agent followed by close monitoring. Either oral or intravenous N-acetylcysteine should be given to patients with a history of acetaminophen poisoning. For those patients who develop acute liver failure due to nonacetaminophen drugs, one study demonstrated a benefit with intravenous N-acetylcysteine.[33]

KEY POINTS

- Most reports of DILI in pregnancy involve antiretroviral therapy and alpha-methyldopa.
- Primary treatment is withdrawal of the offending medication.

DISEASES UNIQUE TO PREGNANCY

HYPEREMESIS GRAVIDARUM

Hyperemesis gravidarum (HG) is defined as intractable vomiting associated with weight loss of greater than 5% of prepregnancy weight and ketonuria.[34] The cause of this condition is unclear, but it is likely multifactorial and may include hormonal, psychological, and genetic factors.[35] Incidence estimates vary between 0.5% and 2% of pregnancies.[36,37] Patients typically present early in the first trimester of pregnancy with persistent nausea and vomiting, and the symptoms usually resolve during the second trimester. As opposed to the more common and mild nausea and vomiting of pregnancy, patients with HG usually require hospitalization for intravenous hydration. Abnormal serum liver chemistries have been reported in 16% of patients hospitalized for HG.[38] Moderate elevation in the aminotransferases (up to 4 times the upper limit of normal) is seen predominantly; hyperbilirubinemia and jaundice can be found less commonly. More severe transaminitis (greater than 1000 IU/L) can also be observed rarely.[39] The cause of these lab abnormalities is unknown. In addition to the abnormal liver tests, electrolyte abnormalities and elevations in the urea nitrogen are common, owing to volume depletion. Hyperthyroidism is often seen in this condition as well, possibly due to the thyroid-stimulating activity of human chorionic gonadotropin.[40] The diagnosis of HG is made on clinical grounds alone; liver biopsy is usually not required, but if performed can show nonspecific changes including mild steatosis and cholestasis. There are no liver-specific therapies for this condition. Treatment of patients with HG includes intravenous hydration and bowel rest initially. Thiamine supplementation should be provided to prevent the development of Wernicke's encephalopathy, which has been reported as a complication of HG.[41] Antiemetics should be used, but data are insufficient to recommend one class of antiemetics over another.[35] Glucocorticoids have also been used in patients with refractory symptoms, but a randomized, placebo-controlled trial demonstrated no benefit.[42] Support with enteral or parenteral nutrition is required for those with symptoms refractory to pharmacologic therapy; enteral feeding is preferred given the infectious risks associated with parenteral nutrition. Low birth weight, preterm delivery, and birth defects are no more likely in patients with HG compared to the general population.[43] Liver-related complications have not been reported.

KEY POINTS
• Patients with HG present in the first trimester with persistent nausea and vomiting.
• Abnormal liver chemistries are common in the setting of HG, but liver-related complications do not occur.

INTRAHEPATIC CHOLESTASIS OF PREGNANCY

Intrahepatic cholestasis of pregnancy (ICP) refers to the onset of pruritus associated with elevated serum bile acids during the second half of pregnancy with resolution following delivery.[44] The incidence of ICP varies widely between regions. The highest known frequency is in Chile, where up to 15.6% of pregnancies have been affected, with substantial variation between ethnic groups.[45] It has been reported in up to 1.5% of pregnancies in Sweden.[44] In the United States, incidence reports have varied between 0.32% and 5.6% depending on the group studied.[46,47] The etiology appears to be multifactorial, involving genetic and hormonal factors. Multiple studies have highlighted the importance of genetic mutations in canalicular bile salt and phospholipid transporters in the disease pathogenesis.[48,49] In addition, estrogen is known to be a cholestatic hormone,[50] and exogenous progesterone administration is associated with an increased risk of ICP,[51] suggesting a contributory role for female sex hormones. The incidence of ICP is also increased in multiple gestation pregnancies, which are associated with higher levels of circulating estrogen.[52] Despite these associations, an exact cause for this condition is not known.

The hallmark symptom of ICP is generalized pruritus, which can be quite severe. Particular involvement of the palms and soles can be seen. Jaundice occurs in less than 10% of patients and typically follows the onset of pruritus by weeks. Jaundice without pruritus is exceedingly rare.[51] Encephalopathy and other signs of liver failure do not occur and should prompt an evaluation for alternate causes of ALI. Physical examination can show excoriations due to scratching. Fasting bile acids are invariably elevated (by definition), and other cholestatic laboratory values can be seen. The bilirubin is usually less than 5 mg/dL.[51] Unlike other cholestatic conditions, the GGT is usually less than twice the upper limit of normal. Aminotransferases are typically elevated as well and can be greater than 1000 IU/L. A prolonged prothrombin time reflects vitamin K deficiency due to cholestasis and not liver dysfunction. Ultrasound examination of the liver is normal. Liver biopsy is generally not needed for the diagnosis, but if performed, it will show cholestasis without inflammation or necrosis and preserved portal tracts.

In the absence of other risk factors for liver disease, maternal outcomes are favorable. However, in one large population-based cohort study, women with ICP did have an increased risk of hepatitis C, nonalcoholic liver cirrhosis, and gallstone disease.[53] Therefore, women with ICP should be screened for chronic viral hepatitis and should be followed postpartum to ensure normalization of liver biochemical tests. Most women with ICP will have recurrent cholestasis in subsequent pregnancies. Much of the morbidity associated with ICP is related to fetal outcomes, particularly when the serum bile acid concentration is greater than 40 μmol/L.[44] The risk of preterm labor is increased compared to the general population, with wide variability in the reported incidence.[44,51] Neonates are also at increased risk for the development of respiratory distress syndrome, possibly related to the presence of bile acids in the lungs.[54] The risk of intrauterine fetal demise is also increased and has been reported in up to 5% of pregnancies.[51,55] The cause is unknown. Fetal demise typically occurs in the last month of pregnancy, and routine antenatal monitoring is not predictive of a poor outcome.[55]

The focus of treatment is symptom reduction and the prevention of neonatal morbidity. Ursodeoxycholic acid (UDCA) at a dose of 15 mg/kg/day has been shown to reduce pruritus and to improve some fetal outcomes in multiple studies,[56,57] and it is currently recommended for treatment of ICP. The mechanism by which UDCA benefits patients is not entirely clear but is likely related to its effect on serum bile acid composition, which is altered in patients with ICP.[58] Cholestyramine, a bile salt-binding agent, can be used to decrease ileal absorption of bile salts, but it is less effective than UDCA,[56] can increase steatorrhea, and can exacerbate vitamin K deficiency. Vitamin K deficiency should be identified and corrected parenterally prior to delivery to prevent hemorrhage. The glutathione precursor S-adenosyl-L-methionine (SAMe) has beneficial effects in models of estrogen-induced cholestasis,[59] but is less effective than UDCA for ICP in clinical trials.[60] Although consensus is lacking, many recommend systematic delivery at 37 weeks gestation because most cases of fetal demise occur after this time.[61] The benefit of early delivery in reducing fetal demise must be weighed against the potential for increased interventions and complications; no randomized clinical trials have been performed to evaluate this strategy.

KEY POINTS
• ICP presents in the second half of pregnancy with pruritus and elevated serum bile acids; jaundice is rare.
• Recurrence in subsequent pregnancies is common.
• First-line treatment for ICP is ursodiol.
• Early delivery at 37 weeks may be considered to reduce fetal demise.

PRE-ECLAMPSIA AND HELLP SYNDROME

Pre-eclampsia is defined as new-onset hypertension and pro-teinuria after 20 weeks of gestation. It occurs in 5% to 10% of all pregnancies and can be classified as mild or severe in the pres-ence of other systemic manifestations, such as liver abnormalities. The condition is labeled eclampsia when seizures are present. The pathogenesis of pre-eclampsia is not entirely clear but likely involves abnormal placental development, which induces maternal systemic endothelial dysfunction and subsequent end-organ damage.[62] There are multiple risk factors for the development of pre-eclampsia, the most prominent of which include primiparity, advanced maternal age, medical comorbidities, family history, and pre-eclampsia dur-ing a prior pregnancy.[62] Up to 30% of cases can occur postpartum, typically within 48 hours of delivery.[63] Aside from hypertension and proteinuria, additional clinical features are nonspecific and can include headache, vision changes, dyspnea, nausea and vomit-ing, epigastric pain, oliguria, and edema. Epigastric pain may be the result of stretching of Glisson's capsule from hepatic edema or bleeding. Laboratory evaluation may demonstrate an elevated creatinine, thrombocytopenia, elevation of the serum lactate dehy-drogenase and the presence of schistocytes on a peripheral smear indicative of hemolysis, and aminotransferase elevation. The com-bination of hemolysis, elevated liver enzymes, and low platelets (HELLP), which can occur in up to 20% of patients with severe pre-eclampsia, is thought to be a form of severe pre-eclampsia, though HELLP can occur in the absence of hypertension and pro-teinuria.[63] Aminotransferases can be elevated up to several hundred IU/L. More significant elevations are rare and may indicate hepatic infarction or rupture. Jaundice is uncommon.[63] Prolongation of the prothrombin time may indicate disseminated intravascular coagu-lation, which can occur in 21% of cases of HELLP.[63] Additional complications of HELLP include abruptio placentae, renal failure, pulmonary edema, and retinal detachment.

There is no consensus definition of what level of laboratory abnor-malities constitutes HELLP, though some have advocated a defini-tion including a platelet count <100 x 10^9/L, an AST ≥70 IU/L, an abnormal peripheral blood smear, and an LDH ≥600 IU/L.[64] Liver biopsy is usually not necessary to make the diagnosis and may be ill advised in the setting of significant thrombocytopenia.

When performed, it shows sinusoidal fibrin thrombi associated with periportal and focal parenchymal necrosis. Imaging is also usually not needed for the diagnosis of HELLP or pre-eclampsia but can be helpful when there is a concern for subcapsular hepatic hematoma or hemorrhage. Outcomes for women who develop HELLP are generally good with appropriate obstetrical management but a minority can have significant morbidity, and the mortality rate is 1%[63] (compared to a mortality rate of 6.4 per 10,000 for pre-eclampsia).[65] Liver-related complications of HELLP include subcapsular hematoma and rupture, intraparenchymal hemorrhage, and acute liver failure.[66] The risk of recurrent pre-eclampsia in subsequent pregnancies has been reported to range from 10% to 65% and is dependent on additional risk factors.[67] The risk of recurrent HELLP, however, is low.[68] Neonatal morbidity and mortality is related to prematurity; the overall mortality rate in one study of 308 births was 15%, the majority of which occurred in those delivered prior to 29 weeks gestation.[69] Surviving infants have no increase in morbidity directly attributable to pre-eclampsia.[70]

Patients with HELLP or severe pre-eclampsia should be hospitalized and monitored closely. Coagulopathy should be corrected, and magnesium sulfate should be administered for seizure prophylaxis.[71] Severe hypertension should be treated with hydralazine, labetalol, or nifedipine.[64] In pregnancies remote from term, the patient should be transferred to a center with appropriate neonatal support. After maternal stabilization, fetal monitoring should be instituted. The mainstay of therapy is delivery. Prompt delivery is indicated if the pregnancy is over 34 weeks gestation; if there is evidence of fetal distress; or if there is maternal multiorgan dysfunction, DIC, renal failure, or abruptio placentae.[72] Management of pregnancies remote from term is controversial. For carefully selected women with severe pre-eclampsia, including those with mild aminotransferase abnormalities, delay of delivery (ie, expectant management) can prolong the pregnancy without an increase in maternal or fetal complications.[73] A few studies have shown successful reversal of laboratory abnormalities and prolongation of pregnancy with expectant management in the setting of HELLP[74,75]; however, there is no evidence that overall perinatal outcomes are improved with this approach. In the setting of significant neonatal mortality, many experts do not advocate routine expectant management in this patient population.[64] Prior to 34 weeks gestation, corticosteroids should be given for the promotion of fetal lung maturity; they offer no substantive maternal clinical benefit in the setting of HELLP.[76] The mode of delivery should be individualized. Women with well-established labor may proceed with vaginal birth in the absence of obstetrical contraindications, but C-section should be considered for those with an unripe cervix or before 30 weeks gestation.[64] Following delivery, HELLP usually resolves rapidly.

Liver-specific complications of HELLP include hepatic hematoma and rupture, as well as liver failure. These conditions can carry a very high mortality and may require a multidisciplinary approach to management, including interventional radiology, trauma surgery, and transplant surgery. Initial therapy for these patients is supportive with volume resuscitation and blood transfusion as appropriate. For those patients with hemorrhage without rupture, conservative management may be appropriate with serial imaging and consideration of hepatic artery embolization.[77] Rupture of a hematoma may present with increased abdominal pain, massive ascites, or hemodynamic shock and is a surgical emergency. In this circumstance, primary laparotomy with temporary packing of the liver for control of bleeding is a reasonable approach.[78] Liver transplantation may be an option for patients with uncontrolled hemorrhage or extensive necrosis and subsequent acute liver failure.[79]

KEY POINTS

- Pre-eclampsia presents in the second half of pregnancy with hypertension and proteinuria.
- HELLP syndrome is common in the setting of pre-eclampsia.
- Liver-related complications may include hemorrhage and liver failure.
- Treatment of HELLP is medical stabilization followed by prompt delivery.
- Neonatal morbidity and mortality is related to prematurity.

ACUTE FATTY LIVER OF PREGNANCY

Acute fatty liver of pregnancy (AFLP) is characterized by microvesicular fatty infiltration of hepatocytes during the second half of pregnancy and is a medical emergency. It is a rare disorder with an incidence of 1 per 20,000 deliveries,[80] but its importance is underscored by its historically high maternal mortality rate.[81] The cause of this condition is not entirely understood but it likely relates to defects in mitochondrial β oxidation of fatty acids. The enzyme long-chain 3-hydroxyacyl-CoA dehydrogenase (LCHAD) is a component of the mitochondrial machinery that accomplishes β oxidation in the liver, and both maternal and fetal deficiencies of this enzyme are associated with AFLP.[82,83] Currently, the most accepted hypothesis is that a homozygous LCHAD-deficient fetus will produce toxic long-chain 3-hydroxyacyl metabolites that accumulate and cause liver damage in the heterozygous mother.[84] Later, infants with LCHAD deficiency can present with liver failure, cardiomyopathy, hypoglycemic encephalopathy, or sudden death and are treated with dietary restriction of long-chain fatty acids.[85] Thus, because of the significant association between AFLP and fetal LCHAD deficiency, screening newborns from AFLP-complicated pregnancies for mutations causing LCHAD deficiency is recommended.[86]

Clinically, patients typically present with nonspecific symptoms including nausea, vomiting, abdominal pain, and anorexia. Fever and jaundice are common physical examination findings. The liver itself is usually not palpable.[85] Patients also may present with multisystem involvement, including encephalopathy, gastrointestinal bleeding, coagulopathy, or pancreatitis.[84] Concomitant pre-eclampsia or HELLP are common.[72] The median gestational age is 36 weeks at diagnosis, and patients are almost always beyond 28 weeks gestation.[80] Primiparity and multiple gestation pregnancies appear to be risk factors for the development of AFLP.[80] Various abnormal laboratory values indicate the multisystem dysfunction that can be present with AFLP. Peak aminotransferases are typically several hundred IU/L but can be greater than 1000 IU/L. The bilirubin is often elevated as well. Leukocytosis, thrombocytopenia, and coagulopathy can all be seen. Hypoglycemia is frequently encountered, and the serum creatinine is often increased.[80] Ultrasonography may demonstrate increased echogenicity but imaging is often normal. The diagnosis of AFLP is made on clinical grounds based on characteristic test results in the appropriate clinical setting. Liver biopsy is the gold standard diagnostic test but is rarely needed and is often avoided because of its associated risks. Histologic findings include microvesicular fatty infiltration of hepatocytes in zones 2 and 3 with sparing of the periportal hepatocytes, cholestasis, and mild inflammation. When performing the biopsy, if AFLP is suspected, a piece of the specimen should be reserved for oil red O staining or electron microscopy to confirm the presence of fat in patients without typical hematoxylin and eosin (H & E) findings.[84]

Maternal outcomes have been poor historically, with a mortality rate of 75%.[81] However, with improved recognition and prompt treatment, outcomes have improved drastically. In one large population-based study of 57 women with AFLP, there was only one maternal death.[80] There was significant morbidity, however; 8 women developed renal failure and 4 required intubation. In another series of 32 patients, infectious complications developed in half of the patients, intra-abdominal bleeding was common, and the maternal mortality rate was 12.5%.[87] The neonatal mortality rate has been reported to be 10%.[80] There is no specific medical therapy for AFLP. The primary treatment is delivery, as the condition will not resolve spontaneously. Maternal stabilization should be performed initially with close attention to blood glucose and correction of hypoglycemia as well as coagulopathy, followed by urgent delivery.[84] The majority of women require C-section.[80] Clinical and biochemical improvement typically occur within the first few days postpartum. Liver transplantation has been reported for fulminant liver failure due to AFLP[88] but is typically not necessary with early diagnosis and prompt delivery.[66] Given the rarity of this condition, the risk of recurrent AFLP in subsequent pregnancies is not known but has been reported even in the absence of LCHAD mutations.[89]

KEY POINTS
• AFLP presents with multisystem dysfunction and occurs in the last trimester.
• Improved recognition and prompt treatment have led to better outcomes.
• Treatment involves maternal stabilization followed by urgent delivery.
• Newborns should be screened for LCHAD deficiency mutations.

SUMMARY

Although rare, acute liver disease in pregnancy is an important topic because of the substantial morbidity that can accompany some of these diagnoses. Moreover, early diagnosis and intervention can have a positive impact on clinical outcomes. There are relatively few conditions that cause ALI in pregnancy, and most of these conditions can be differentiated from one another by clinical characteristics as well as laboratory markers. Particular attention should be paid to the patient's symptoms, the gestational age, and the pattern of laboratory test abnormalities. For instance, a woman with debilitating vomiting in the first trimester and abnormal aminotransferases is likely to have HG, whereas the onset of intense pruritus in the third trimester with a slight hyperbilirubinemia probably represents ICP. In addition, non–pregnancy-related causes of ALI must also be considered and should be excluded. It is important to consider the safety of various medications used in the management of ALI in both pregnancy and breastfeeding (see Table 12-2). As discussed in each section, rarely is a liver biopsy needed for diagnostic or management purposes; most diagnoses can be made noninvasively, avoiding the risks associated with biopsy. In any case, when the diagnosis is questionable, referral to a hepatologist may be appropriate to aid in diagnostic testing, decision making, and therapeutic management.

REFERENCES

1. Ch'ng CL, Morgan M, Hainsworth I, Kingham JG. Prospective study of liver dysfunction in pregnancy in Southwest Wales. *Gut.* 2002;51(6):876-880.
2. Gordon MC. Maternal physiology. In: Gabbe SG, Niebyl JR, Simpson JL, eds. *Obstetrics: Normal and Problem Pregnancies.* Vol 5. Philadelphia, PA: Churchill Livingstone Elsevier; 2007:55.
3. Boehlen F, Hohlfeld P, Extermann P, Perneger TV, De Moerloose P. Platelet count at term pregnancy: a reappraisal of the threshold. *Obstetrics & Gynecology.* 2000;95(1):29-33.
4. Adeniyi FA, Olatunbosun DA. Origins and significance of the increased plasma alkaline phosphatase during normal pregnancy and pre-eclampsia. *Br J Obstet Gynaecol.* 1984;91(9):857-862.
5. Bacq Y, Zarka O, Brechot JF, et al. Liver function tests in normal pregnancy: a prospective study of 103 pregnant women and 103 matched controls. *Hepatology (Baltimore, Md).* 1996;23(5):1030-1034.

Table 12-2

Medication Recommendations for Pregnancy and Breastfeeding in Acute Liver Diseases

Medication	FDA Pregnancy Category*	Pregnancy Comment	Breastfeeding Comment
Hepatitis A vaccine	C	Low risk, limited human data	Low risk, no human data
Immune globulin	C	Low risk, limited human data	Low risk, human data
Hepatitis B vaccine	C	Low risk, limited human data	Low risk, no human data
Hepatitis B immune globulin	C	Low risk, limited human data	Low risk, no human data
Heparin	C	Low risk; does not cross placenta; human data	Low risk; does not enter breast milk; no human data
Enoxaparin	B	Low risk; does not cross placenta; human data	Low risk; not detected in nursing infants; limited human data
Dalteparin	B	Low risk; does not cross placenta; limited human data	Low risk; low levels in breast milk; limited human data
Warfarin	X	Contraindicated; teratogenic to humans; human data	Low risk; does not enter breast milk; limited human data
N-acetylcysteine	B	Low risk, human data	Low risk, no human data
Thiamine	A	Essential nutrient, human data	Low risk, no human data

(continued)

Table 12-2 *(continued)*

Medication Recommendations for Pregnancy and Breastfeeding in Acute Liver Diseases

Medication	FDA Pregnancy Category*	Pregnancy Comment	Breastfeeding Comment
UDCA	B	Low risk, limited human data	Low risk; detected in breast milk; limited human data
Vitamin K	C	Low risk, human data	Low risk, limited human data
Hydralazine	C	Low risk, human data	Low risk, limited human data
Labetalol	C	Low risk, human data	Low risk, human data
Nifedipine	C	Low risk, limited human data	Low risk, human data

Adapted from Micromedex Healthcare Series. Thomson Reuters (Healthcare) Inc.; 2011. http://www.thomsonhc.com/micromedex2/librarian/. Accessed July 2011; Reprotox. The Reproductive Toxicology Center; 2011. http://www.reprotox.org/. Accessed July 2011; and LactMed. National Library of Medicine; 2011. http://toxnet.nlm.nih.gov/cgi-bin/sis/htmlgen?LACT. Accessed July 2011.

6. Taylor RM, Davern T, Munoz S, et al. Fulminant hepatitis A virus infection in the United States: Incidence, prognosis, and outcomes. *Hepatology (Baltimore, Md.)*. 2006;44(6):1589-1597.

7. Fiore S, Savasi V. Treatment of viral hepatitis in pregnancy. *Expert Opinion on Pharmacotherapy*. 2009;10(17):2801-2809.

8. Elinav E, Ben-Dov IZ, Shapira Y, et al. Acute hepatitis A infection in pregnancy is associated with high rates of gestational complications and preterm labor. *Gastroenterology*. 2006;130(4):1129-1134.

9. American College of Obstetrics and Gynecologists. ACOG Practice Bulletin No. 86: Viral hepatitis in pregnancy. *Obstet Gynecol*. 2007;110(4):941-956.

10. Tassopoulos NC, Papaevangelou GJ, Sjogren MH, Roumeliotou-Karayannis A, Gerin JL, Purcell RH. Natural history of acute hepatitis B surface antigen-positive hepatitis in Greek adults. *Gastroenterology*. 1987;92(6):1844-1850.

11. Hieber JP, Dalton D, Shorey J, Combes B. Hepatitis and pregnancy. *J Pediatr*. 1977;91(4):545-549.

12. Sookoian S. Liver disease during pregnancy: acute viral hepatitis. *Ann Hepatol.* 2006;5(3):231-236.

13. Mast EE, Margolis HS, Fiore AE, et al. A comprehensive immunization strategy to eliminate transmission of hepatitis B virus infection in the United States: recommendations of the Advisory Committee on Immunization Practices (ACIP) part 1: immunization of infants, children, and adolescents. *MMWR Recommendations and Reports: Morbidity and Mortality Weekly Report.* 2005;54(RR-16):1-31.

14. Lok AS, McMahon BJ. Chronic hepatitis B: update 2009. *Hepatology (Baltimore, Md).* 2009;50(3):661-662.

15. Withers MR, Correa MT, Morrow M, et al. Antibody levels to hepatitis E virus in North Carolina swine workers, non-swine workers, swine, and murids. *Am J Tropical Med Hygiene.* 2002;66(4):384-388.

16. Khuroo MS, Teli MR, Skidmore S, Sofi MA, Khuroo MI. Incidence and severity of viral hepatitis in pregnancy. *Am J Med.* 1981;70(2):252-255.

17. Patra S, Kumar A, Trivedi SS, Puri M, Sarin SK. Maternal and fetal outcomes in pregnant women with acute hepatitis E virus infection. *Ann Intern Med.* 2007;147(1):28-33.

18. Kar P, Jilani N, Husain SA, et al. Does hepatitis E viral load and genotypes influence the final outcome of acute liver failure during pregnancy? *Am J Gastroenterol.* 2008;103(10):2495-2501.

19. Khuroo MS, Kamili S. Clinical course and duration of viremia in vertically transmitted hepatitis E virus (HEV) infection in babies born to HEV-infected mothers. *J Viral Hepatitis.* 2009;16(7):519-523.

20. Zhu FC, Zhang J, Zhang XF, et al. Efficacy and safety of a recombinant hepatitis E vaccine in healthy adults: a large-scale, randomised, double-blind placebo-controlled, phase 3 trial. *Lancet.* 2010;376(9744):895-902.

21. Darwish Murad S, Plessier A, Hernandez-Guerra M, et al. Etiology, management, and outcome of the Budd-Chiari syndrome. *Ann Intern Med.* 2009;151(3):167-175.

22. Rautou PE, Moucari R, Cazals-Hatem D, et al. Levels and initial course of serum alanine aminotransferase can predict outcome of patients with Budd-Chiari syndrome. *Clin Gastroenterol Hepatol.* 2009;7(11):1230-1235.

23. Rautou PE, Plessier A, Bernuau J, Denninger MH, Moucari R, Valla D. Pregnancy: a risk factor for Budd-Chiari syndrome? *Gut.* 2009;58(4):606-608.

24. DeLeve LD, Valla DC, Garcia-Tsao G, American Association for the Study Liver Disease. Vascular disorders of the liver. *Hepatology (Baltimore, Md).* 2009;49(5):1729-1764.

25. Garcia-Pagan JC, Heydtmann M, Raffa S, et al. TIPS for Budd-Chiari syndrome: long-term results and prognostics factors in 124 patients. *Gastroenterology.* 2008;135(3):808-815.

26. Buchel E, Van Steenbergen W, Nevens F, Fevery J. Improvement of autoimmune hepatitis during pregnancy followed by flare-up after delivery. *Am J Gastroenterol.* 2002;97(12):3160-3165.

27. Ostapowicz G, Fontana RJ, Schiodt FV, et al. Results of a prospective study of acute liver failure at 17 tertiary care centers in the United States. *Ann Intern Med.* 2002;137(12):947-954.

28. Watkins PB, Seeff LB. Drug-induced liver injury: summary of a single topic clinical research conference. *Hepatology (Baltimore, Md)*. 2006;43(3): 618-631.

29. Bjornsson E. Drug-induced liver injury: Hy's rule revisited. *Clin Pharmacol Therapeutics*. 2006;79(6):521-528.

30. Phanuphak N, Apornpong T, Teeratakulpisarn S, et al. Nevirapine-associated toxicity in HIV-infected Thai men and women, including pregnant women. *HIV Medicine*. 2007;8(6):357-366.

31. Slim R, Ben Salem C, Hmouda H, Bouraoui K. Hepatotoxicity of alpha-methyldopa in pregnancy. *J Clinical Pharm Therapeutics*. 2010;35(3):361-363.

32. Hill JB, Sheffield JS, Zeeman GG, Wendel GD Jr. Hepatotoxicity with antiretroviral treatment of pregnant women. *Obstet Gynecol*. 2001;98(5 Pt 2):909-911.

33. Lee WM, Hynan LS, Rossaro L, et al. Intravenous N-acetylcysteine improves transplant-free survival in early stage non-acetaminophen acute liver failure. *Gastroenterology*. 2009;137(3):856-864, 864.e851.

34. Goodwin TM. Hyperemesis gravidarum. *Clin Obstet Gynecology*. 1998;41(3):597-605.

35. Sanu O, Lamont RF. Hyperemesis gravidarum: pathogenesis and the use of antiemetic agents. *Expert Opinion on Pharmacotherapy*. 2011;12(5):737-748.

36. Kallen B. Hyperemesis during pregnancy and delivery outcome: a registry study. *Eur Journal Obstet, Gynecol, Reproductive Biol*. 1987;26(4):291-302.

37. Bailit JL. Hyperemesis gravidarum: Epidemiologic findings from a large cohort. *Am J Obstet Gynecol*. 2005;193(3 Pt 1):811-814.

38. Morali GA, Braverman DZ. Abnormal liver enzymes and ketonuria in hyperemesis gravidarum. A retrospective review of 80 patients. *J Clin Gastroenterol*. 1990;12(3):303-305.

39. Conchillo JM, Pijnenborg JM, Peeters P, Stockbrugger RW, Fevery J, Koek GH. Liver enzyme elevation induced by hyperemesis gravidarum: aetiology, diagnosis and treatment. *The Netherlands J Med*. 2002;60(9):374-378.

40. Goodwin TM, Montoro M, Mestman JH, Pekary AE, Hershman JM. The role of chorionic gonadotropin in transient hyperthyroidism of hyperemesis gravidarum. *J Clin Endocrinol Metabolism*. 1992;75(5):1333-1337.

41. Chiossi G, Neri I, Cavazzuti M, Basso G, Facchinetti F. Hyperemesis gravidarum complicated by Wernicke encephalopathy: background, case report, and review of the literature. *Obstet Gynecol Surv*. 2006;61(4):255-268.

42. Yost NP, McIntire DD, Wians FH Jr, Ramin SM, Balko JA, Leveno KJ. A randomized, placebo-controlled trial of corticosteroids for hyperemesis due to pregnancy. *Obstet Gynecol*. 2003;102(6):1250-1254.

43. Tsang IS, Katz VL, Wells SD. Maternal and fetal outcomes in hyperemesis gravidarum. *Int J Gynaecol Obstet*. 1996;55(3):231-235.

44. Glantz A, Marschall HU, Mattsson LA. Intrahepatic cholestasis of pregnancy: relationships between bile acid levels and fetal complication rates. *Hepatology (Baltimore, Md)*. 2004;40(2):467-474.

45. Reyes H, Gonzalez MC, Ribalta J, et al. Prevalence of intrahepatic cholestasis of pregnancy in Chile. *Ann Intern Med*. 1978;88(4):487-493.

46. Laifer SA, Stiller RJ, Siddiqui DS, Dunston-Boone G, Whetham JC. Ursodeoxycholic acid for the treatment of intrahepatic cholestasis of pregnancy. *J Maternal-Fetal Med*. 2001;10(2):131-135.

47. Lee RH, Goodwin TM, Greenspoon J, Incerpi M. The prevalence of intrahepatic cholestasis of pregnancy in a primarily Latina Los Angeles population. *J Perinatol.* 2006;26(9):527-532.
48. Dixon PH, van Mil SW, Chambers J, et al. Contribution of variant alleles of ABCB11 to susceptibility to intrahepatic cholestasis of pregnancy. *Gut.* 2009;58(4):537-544.
49. Mullenbach R, Bennett A, Tetlow N, et al. ATP8B1 mutations in British cases with intrahepatic cholestasis of pregnancy. *Gut.* 2005;54(6):829-834.
50. Kern F Jr, Eriksson H, Curstedt T, Sjovall J. Effect of ethynylestradiol on biliary excretion of bile acids, phosphatidylcolines, and cholesterol in the bile fistula rat. *J Lipid Res.* 1977;18(5):623-634.
51. Bacq Y, Sapey T, Brechot MC, Pierre F, Fignon A, Dubois F. Intrahepatic cholestasis of pregnancy: a French prospective study. *Hepatology (Baltimore, Md).* 1997;26(2):358-364.
52. Gonzalez MC, Reyes H, Arrese M, et al. Intrahepatic cholestasis of pregnancy in twin pregnancies. *J Hepatol.* 1989;9(1):84-90.
53. Ropponen A, Sund R, Riikonen S, Ylikorkala O, Aittomaki K. Intrahepatic cholestasis of pregnancy as an indicator of liver and biliary diseases: a population-based study. *Hepatology (Baltimore, Md).* 2006;43(4):723-728.
54. Zecca E, De Luca D, Baroni S, Vento G, Tiberi E, Romagnoli C. Bile acid-induced lung injury in newborn infants: a bronchoalveolar lavage fluid study. *Pediatrics.* 2008;121(1):e146-149.
55. Alsulyman OM, Ouzounian JG, Ames-Castro M, Goodwin TM. Intrahepatic cholestasis of pregnancy: perinatal outcome associated with expectant management. *Am J Obstet Gynecol.* 1996;175(4 Pt 1):957-960.
56. Kondrackiene J, Beuers U, Kupcinskas L. Efficacy and safety of ursodeoxycholic acid versus cholestyramine in intrahepatic cholestasis of pregnancy. *Gastroenterology.* 2005;129(3):894-901.
57. Glantz A, Marschall HU, Lammert F, Mattsson LA. Intrahepatic cholestasis of pregnancy: a randomized controlled trial comparing dexamethasone and ursodeoxycholic acid. *Hepatology (Baltimore, Md).* 2005;42(6):1399-1405.
58. Brites D, Rodrigues CM, Oliveira N, Cardoso M, Graca LM. Correction of maternal serum bile acid profile during ursodeoxycholic acid therapy in cholestasis of pregnancy. *J Hepatol.* 1998;28(1):91-98.
59. Stramentinoli G, Di Padova C, Gualano M, Rovagnati P, Galli-Kienle M. Ethynylestradiol-induced impairment of bile secretion in the rat: protective effects of S-adenosyl-L-methionine and its implication in estrogen metabolism. *Gastroenterology.* 1981;80(1):154-158.
60. Binder T, Salaj P, Zima T, Vitek L. Randomized prospective comparative study of ursodeoxycholic acid and S-adenosyl-L-methionine in the treatment of intrahepatic cholestasis of pregnancy. *J Perinatal Med.* 2006;34(5):383-391.
61. Roncaglia N, Arreghini A, Locatelli A, Bellini P, Andreotti C, Ghidini A. Obstetric cholestasis: outcome with active management. *Eur J Obstet, Gynecology, and Reproductive Biol.* 2002;100(2):167-170.
62. Steegers EA, von Dadelszen P, Duvekot JJ, Pijnenborg R. Pre-eclampsia. *Lancet.* 2010;376(9741):631-644.

63. Sibai BM, Ramadan MK, Usta I, Salama M, Mercer BM, Friedman SA. Maternal morbidity and mortality in 442 pregnancies with hemolysis, elevated liver enzymes, and low platelets (HELLP syndrome). *Am J Obstet Gynecol.* 1993;169(4):1000-1006.

64. Barton JR, Sibai BM. Gastrointestinal complications of pre-eclampsia. *Semin Perinatol.* 2009;33(3):179-188.

65. MacKay AP, Berg CJ, Atrash HK. Pregnancy-related mortality from pre-eclampsia and eclampsia. *Obstetr Gynecol.* 2001;97(4):533-538.

66. Westbrook RH, Yeoman AD, Joshi D, et al. Outcomes of severe pregnancy-related liver disease: refining the role of transplantation. *Am J Transplantation.* 2010;10(11):2520-2526.

67. Barton JR, Sibai BM. Prediction and prevention of recurrent preeclampsia. *Obstet Gynecol.* 2008;112(2 Pt 1):359-372.

68. Sibai BM, Ramadan MK, Chari RS, Friedman SA. Pregnancies complicated by HELLP syndrome (hemolysis, elevated liver enzymes, and low platelets): subsequent pregnancy outcome and long-term prognosis. *Am J Obstet Gynecol.* 1995;172(1 Pt 1):125-129.

69. Sibai BM, Spinnato JA, Watson DL, Hill GA, Anderson GD. Pregnancy outcome in 303 cases with severe preeclampsia. *Obstet Gynecol.* 1984;64(3):319-325.

70. Harms K, Rath W, Herting E, Kuhn W. Maternal hemolysis, elevated liver enzymes, low platelet count, and neonatal outcome. *Am J Perinatol.* 1995;12(1):1-6.

71. Witlin AG, Sibai BM. Magnesium sulfate therapy in preeclampsia and eclampsia. *Obstet Gynecol.* 1998;92(5):883-889.

72. Hay JE. Liver disease in pregnancy. *Hepatology (Baltimore, Md).* 2008;47(3): 1067-1076.

73. Magee LA, Yong PJ, Espinosa V, Cote AM, Chen I, von Dadelszen P. Expectant management of severe preeclampsia remote from term: a structured systematic review. *Hypertension in Pregnancy.* 2009;28(3):312-347.

74. Visser W, Wallenburg HC. Temporising management of severe pre-eclampsia with and without the HELLP syndrome. *Br J Obstet Gynaecol.* 1995;102(2): 111-117.

75. van Pampus MG, Wolf H, Westenberg SM, van der Post JA, Bonsel GJ, Treffers PE. Maternal and perinatal outcome after expectant management of the HELLP syndrome compared with pre-eclampsia without HELLP syndrome. *Eur J Obstet, Gynecol, Reproductive Biol.* 1998;76(1):31-36.

76. Woudstra DM, Chandra S, Hofmeyr GJ, Dowswell T. Corticosteroids for HELLP (hemolysis, elevated liver enzymes, low platelets) syndrome in pregnancy. *Cochrane Database of Systematic Reviews (Online).* 2010;(9)(9): CD008148.

77. Rinehart BK, Terrone DA, Magann EF, Martin RW, May WL, Martin JN Jr. Preeclampsia-associated hepatic hemorrhage and rupture: mode of management related to maternal and perinatal outcome. *Obstet Gynecol Surv.* 1999;54(3):196-202.

78. Reck T, Bussenius-Kammerer M, Ott R, Muller V, Beinder E, Hohenberger W. Surgical treatment of HELLP syndrome-associated liver rupture—an update. *Eur J Obstetrics, Gynecol, Reproductive Biol.* 2001;99(1):57-65.

79. Shames BD, Fernandez LA, Sollinger HW, et al. Liver transplantation for HELLP syndrome. *Liver Transplantation.* 2005;11(2):224-228.

80. Knight M, Nelson-Piercy C, Kurinczuk JJ, Spark P, Brocklehurst P, System UKOS. A prospective national study of acute fatty liver of pregnancy in the UK. *Gut.* 2008;57(7):951-956.

81. Varner M, Rinderknecht NK. Acute fatty metamorphosis of pregnancy. A maternal mortality and literature review. *J Reproductive Med.* 1980;24(4):177-180.

82. Treem WR, Shoup ME, Hale DE, et al. Acute fatty liver of pregnancy, hemolysis, elevated liver enzymes, and low platelets syndrome, and long chain 3-hydroxyacyl-coenzyme A dehydrogenase deficiency. *Am J Gastroenterol.* 1996;91(11):2293-2300.

83. Ibdah JA, Bennett MJ, Rinaldo P, et al. A fetal fatty-acid oxidation disorder as a cause of liver disease in pregnant women. *N Engl J Med.* 1999;340(22):1723-1731.

84. Bacq Y. Liver diseases unique to pregnancy: a 2010 update. *Clin Res Hepatol Gastroenterol.* 2011;35(3):182-193.

85. Ko H, Yoshida EM. Acute fatty liver of pregnancy. *Can J Gastroenterol.* 2006;20(1):25-30.

86. Yang Z, Yamada J, Zhao Y, Strauss AW, Ibdah JA. Prospective screening for pediatric mitochondrial trifunctional protein defects in pregnancies complicated by liver disease. *JAMA.* 2002;288(17):2163-2166.

87. Pereira SP, O'Donohue J, Wendon J, Williams R. Maternal and perinatal outcome in severe pregnancy-related liver disease. *Hepatology (Baltimore, Md).* 1997;26(5):1258-1262.

88. Ockner SA, Brunt EM, Cohn SM, Krul ES, Hanto DW, Peters MG. Fulminant hepatic failure caused by acute fatty liver of pregnancy treated by orthotopic liver transplantation. *Hepatology (Baltimore, Md).* 1990;11(1):59-64.

89. Bacq Y, Assor P, Gendrot C, Perrotin F, Scotto B, Andres C. Recurrent acute fatty liver of pregnancy. *Gastroenterologie Clinique et Biologique.* 2007;31(12):1135-1138.

90. Micromedex Healthcare Series. Thomson Reuters (Healthcare) Inc.; 2011. http://www.thomsonhc.com/micromedex2/librarian/. Accessed July 2011.

91. Reprotox. The Reproductive Toxicology Center; 2011. http://www.reprotox.org/. Accessed July 2011.

92. LactMed. National Library of Medicine; 2011. http://toxnet.nlm.nih.gov/cgi-bin/sis/htmlgen?LACT. Accessed July 2011.

Appendix

Classification of Medications During Pregnancy

This book references categories ranging from A to X developed by the Federal Drug Administration (FDA) for use of medications during pregnancy. This classification system has been in effect since 1975. More recently, the FDA began to revamp the drug labeling system by replacing the letter categories with more descriptive and detailed information. This newer system will be used in place of the older categorized system of A to X in the future. This book references the older system due to familiarity, but readers should also be aware of the upcoming changes to pregnancy and lactation drug labeling.[1-3]

THE LETTER CATEGORIZATION SYSTEM

- Category A: Adequate, well-controlled studies have failed to demonstrate risk to the fetus in the first trimester of pregnancy, and there is lack of evidence of risk during the second and third trimesters of pregnancy.

Isaacs KL, Long MD.
*GI and Liver Disease During Pregnancy:
A Practical Approach (pp. 211-216).*
© 2013 Taylor & Francis Group

- Category B: Studies in animals have failed to demonstrate risk to the fetus, and there are no adequate, well-controlled human studies during pregnancy.

- Category C: Animal studies have demonstrated an adverse effect on the fetus, and there are no adequate, well-controlled human studies, but use of the drug during pregnancy may be warranted if the potential benefits are greater than the potential risks with use during pregnancy.

- Category D: Evidence of significant human fetal risk based upon adverse reaction data from investigational or marketing studies in humans, but the potential benefits may outweigh the potential risks for use during pregnancy.

- Category X: Animal or human studies demonstrate fetal abnormalities and/or positive evidence of human fetal risk based on data from investigational or marketing studies, and the risks of using the drug outweigh any potential benefit of use of the drug during pregnancy.

Because the categories may mislead health care providers and pregnant women to believe that risk increases from Category A to B to C to D to X, the system has been redesigned. The new proposed FDA rule would remove the categories from the labeling of all drug products and instead provide a structured narrative. This narrative will provide information in pregnancy and lactation subsections with 3 principal components: a risk summary, a clinical considerations section, and a data section.

The new structured narrative classification system includes sections on pregnancy (with labor and delivery) and lactation.

PREGNANCY SUBSECTION

FETAL RISK SUMMARY

The fetal risk summary will begin with a one-sentence risk conclusion that characterizes the likelihood that the drug increases the risk of 4 types of developmental abnormalities: structural anomalies, fetal and infant mortality, impaired physiologic function, and alterations to growth. An example of a risk conclusion based on human data is as follows: "Human data do not indicate that

Drug X increases the overall risk of structural anomalies." Many of the risk conclusions in the proposed rule are standardized statements that must be used.

The risk conclusion will state whether it is based on animal or human data. More than one risk conclusion may be needed to characterize the likelihood of risk for different developmental abnormalities, doses, durations of exposure, or gestational ages at exposure.

If there are only animal data, the fetal risk summary would contain only the risk conclusion. However, when there are human data, the risk conclusion would be followed by a section describing the most important data about the effects of the drug on the fetus.

CLINICAL CONSIDERATIONS

The clinical considerations component will address 3 main topics important when counseling women who are pregnant, lactating, or of childbearing age: inadvertent exposure, prescribing decisions for pregnant women, and labor and delivery.

Inadvertent Exposure

This section will describe known or predicted risks to the fetus from exposure to the drug early in pregnancy before a woman knows she is pregnant, including data on dose, timing, and duration of exposure.

Prescribing Decisions for Pregnant Women

- Risk to the pregnant woman and the fetus from the disease the drug is indicated to treat
- Dosing adjustments during pregnancy
- Adverse reactions unique to pregnancy associated with use of the drug
- Any interventions that may be needed (eg, monitoring blood glucose for a drug that causes hyperglycemia in pregnancy)
- Any complications in the neonate associated with drug use, including severity, reversibility, and interventions needed

Labor and Delivery

For a drug with a recognized use during labor or delivery (whether or not the drug is indicated for that use), information will be included about the following:

- Effect of the drug on the mother and the fetus/neonate
- Duration of labor and delivery
- Possibility of complications, including needed interventions and the later growth, development, and functional maturation of the child

DATA

The data section will have a more detailed discussion of available data. Human data will appear before animal data. The section will include the following:

- A description of the types of studies
- Animal species used
- Dose exposure information (animal doses described in terms of human dose equivalents)
- Nature of any identified fetal developmental anomalies and other adverse events
- For animal data, an explanation of what is known about the relationship between drug exposure and mechanism of action in animals versus humans

LACTATION SUBSECTION

RISK SUMMARY

If appropriate, this section will include a statement that the use of the drug is compatible with breastfeeding.

- Effects of the drug on milk production
- Whether the drug is present in human milk (and, if so, how much)
- The effect of the drug on the breastfed child

CLINICAL CONSIDERATIONS

- Ways to minimize exposure to the breastfed child, such as timing or pumping and discarding milk

- Potential drug effects in the child and recommendations for monitoring or responding to these effects
- Dosing adjustment during lactation

DATA

Overview of data on which risk summary and clinical considerations are based.

REFERENCES

1. Proposed FDA rule on the federal register, http://www.gpo.gov/fdsys/pkg/FR-2008-05-29/pdf/E8-11806.pdf. Accessed April 24, 2012.
2. Koren G, Sakaguchi S, Klieger C, et al. Toward improved pregnancy labelling. *J Popul Ther Clin Pharmacol.* 2010;17:e349-e357.
3. Briggs GG, Freeman RK, Yaffe SJ. *Drugs in Pregnancy and Lactation: A Reference Guide to Fetal and Neonatal Risk.* 8th ed. Philadelphia, PA: Lippincott Williams & Wilkins, 2008.

Financial Disclosures

Dr. A. Sidney Barritt IV has no financial or proprietary interest in the materials presented herein.

Dr. Spencer D. Dorn has not disclosed any relevant financial relationships.

Dr. Lisa M. Gangarosa has no financial or proprietary interest in the materials presented herein.

Dr. Kim L. Isaacs receives research support from Millenium, GSK, Jannsen, UCB, Abbott, Given, Elan Data Safety Monitoring Board – Jannsen.

Dr. Lindsay E. Jones has not disclosed any relevant financial relationships.

Dr. Patricia D. Jones has no financial or proprietary interest in the materials presented herein.

Dr. Sunanda Kane has not disclosed any relevant financial relationships.

Dr. Millie D. Long has no financial or proprietary interest in the materials presented herein.

Dr. Ryan D. Madanick has no financial or proprietary interest in the materials presented herein.

Dr. Eric S. Orman has no financial or proprietary interest in the materials presented herein.

Dr. D. Wayne Overby has no financial or proprietary interest in the materials presented herein.

Dr. Caitlyn M. Patrick has no financial or proprietary interest in the materials presented herein.

Dr. Megan Quintana has no financial or proprietary interest in the materials presented herein.

Dr. Reza Rahbar has not disclosed any relevant financial relationships.

Dr. Yolanda V. Scarlett has no financial or proprietary interest in the materials presented herein.

Dr. Laurie-Anne C. Swaby has not disclosed any relevant financial relationships.

Index

abdominal pain, 39–60
  biliary colic, 163
  differential diagnosis of, 57–58
  evaluation of, 40–41, 57–58
  gastrointestinal causes of, 43–48
  genitourinary causes of, 50–51
  gynecologic causes of, 53–54
  hepatobiliary causes of, 48–50
  infectious causes of, 54–56
  in irritable bowel syndrome, 82,
    84–85, 87–88
  pregnancy-related causes of, 41–43
  related to physiologic changes, 40
  right lower, differential diagnosis,
    138–139
  vascular causes of, 51–52
acetaminophen poisoning, 194
N-acetylcysteine, for liver disease, 204
acupressure, for nausea and vomiting, 22
acute liver disease, 185–210
  acute fatty liver of pregnancy, 187,
    200–202
  autoimmune hepatitis, 193
  Budd-Chiari syndrome, 192–193
  drug-induced, 193–194
  HELLP syndrome, 187, 198–200
  hepatitis B, 190
  hepatitis E, 191
  hyperemesis gravidarum, 194–195
  intrahepatic cholestasis of pregnan-
    cy, 187, 195–197
  vs. normal pregnancy physiology,
    185
  pre-eclampsia, 187, 198–200

  symptoms of, 188–189
  types of, 186–188
  unique to pregnancy, 194–202
adalimumab, for inflammatory bowel disease, 99, 103
adenomas, hepatic, 50
adnexal masses, 53
alcohol use, pancreatitis in, 161
alternative medicine, for nausea and vomiting, 22
American Society for Gastrointestinal
  Endoscopy guidelines, 117–118
aminosalicylates, for inflammatory bowel
  disease, 96–97, 99
amoxicillin/clavulanate, for inflammatory
  bowel disease, 98
ampicillin, preoperative, 140
ampicillin/sulbactam
  for endoscopy, 125
  for pancreatitis, 156
amylase, in pancreatitis, 49
analgesia
  for endoscopy, 122–127
  for pancreatitis, 155
aneurysm, splenic artery, 53
antacids
  for GERD, 3–4
  for nausea and vomiting, 21
antibiotics
  for endoscopy, 125
  for inflammatory bowel disease,
    97–100
  for pancreatitis, 156

anticholinergics, for nausea and vomiting, 19–20
antidepressants, for irritable bowel syndrome, 84, 87
antihistamines, for nausea and vomiting, 19–20
antispasmodics, for diarrhea, 83–84
appendicitis, 43–44, 136–139
autoimmune hepatitis
      acute, 193
      chronic, 177
azathioprine
      for inflammatory bowel disease, 98, 101–102
      for liver disease, 171, 177

balsalazide, for inflammatory bowel disease, 97
bariatric surgery. *See* gastric bypass
biliary cirrhosis, primary, 178
biliary colic, 163
biliary sludge, 162
biliary tract diseases, 141–145, 161–164
biologic therapy, for inflammatory bowel disease, 98–99, 102–104
bisacodyl, for constipation, 65–67, 86
bismuth subsalicylate, for diarrhea, 83, 87
bladder, infections of, 55
bowel obstruction, 44–45
bowel preparation, for endoscopy, 121–122
breastfeeding
      in GERD, 9
      in inflammatory bowel disease, 95–96, 100–104
      in liver disease, 169–172
      medications used in, 214–215
      in pancreatitis, 155–158
Budd-Chiari syndrome, 186, 192–193

calcitonin, for pancreatitis, 158, 161
calculi, kidney, 50–51
cancer, colorectal, 148–149
castor oil, for constipation, 66–67, 86
cephalosporins
      for endoscopy, 125
      for inflammatory bowel disease, 98, 100
      preoperative, 140
certolizumab pegol, for inflammatory bowel disease, 99, 103–104
chewing gum, for GERD, 7–8
cholangitis, 145
cholecystectomy, 144–145
cholecystitis, 48–49, 143–145, 163
cholecystostomy tube, 145
choledocholithiasis, 145, 163–164

cholestasis, in intrahepatic cholestasis of pregnancy, 187, 195–197
cholestyramine
      for diarrhea, 84, 87
      for liver disease, 197
chronic liver disease, 167–183
      autoimmune hepatitis, 177
      cirrhosis, 168, 173–174
      hepatitis B, 174–175
      hepatitis C, 175–176
      liver transplantation and, 180
      nonalcoholic steatohepatitis, 179
      portal hypertension, 168, 173–174
      primary biliary cirrhosis, 178
      treatment of, 169–172
      Wilson's disease, 178–179
cimetidine, for GERD, 4, 6
ciprofloxacin, for endoscopy, 125
cirrhosis, 168, 173–174
      primary biliary, 178
cisapride, for GERD, 5
cognitive behavioral therapy, for irritable bowel syndrome, 85
colic, biliary, 163
colitis, ulcerative. *See* inflammatory bowel disease
colon, obstruction of, 44–45, 145–146
colon prep solutions, for endoscopy, 129
colonoscopy. *See* endoscopy
colorectal cancer, 148–149
colostomy, for inflammatory bowel disease, 107
complementary and alternative medicine, for nausea and vomiting, 22
computed tomography
      for appendicitis, 137–138
      for inflammatory bowel disease, 105
constipation, 61–73
      criteria for, 61–62
      etiologies of, 61–62
      hemorrhoids in, 68–71, 147–148
      incidence of, 61
      in irritable bowel syndrome, 80, 83, 86
      management of, 65–68
      work-up of, 63–65
copper accumulation, in Wilson's disease, 178
corticosteroids
      for inflammatory bowel disease, 97, 100–101
      for liver disease, 171, 177
      for nausea and vomiting, 21
counseling
      on cirrhosis, 168
      on GERD medications, 9

on inflammatory bowel disease, 92–93
on irritable bowel syndrome, 85
Crohn's disease. *See* inflammatory bowel disease
cyclosporine
 for inflammatory bowel disease, 98, 102
 for liver disease, 172, 180
cystitis, 55

D-penicillamine, for liver disease, 171, 178–179
dalteparin, for liver disease, 204
diabetes, gestational, gastric bypass and, 35
diarrhea, in irritable bowel syndrome, 80–81, 83–84, 87
diazepam
 for endoscopy, 124
 for pancreatitis, 157
dicyclomine, for diarrhea, 83, 87
diet. *See also* nutrition
 for irritable bowel syndrome, 82
 for nausea and vomiting, 18
dimenhydrinate, for nausea and vomiting, 19, 27
diphenhydramine, for nausea and vomiting, 19, 27
diverticulitis, 46
docusate, for constipation, 65–67, 86
dopamine antagonists, for nausea and vomiting, 20
doxylamine-pyridoxine, for nausea and vomiting, 19, 27
droperidol, for nausea and vomiting, 28
drugs. *See* medications

eclampsia, 198–200
embolism, pulmonary, 51–52
endoscopic retrograde cholangiopancreatography, 117, 130, 160
endoscopy, 117–132
 bowel preparation for, 121–122
 electrocautery during, 130
 endoscopic retrograde cholangiopancreatography, 130
 guidelines for, 117–118
 indications for, 118–119
 for inflammatory bowel disease, 106–107
 medications used in, 122–129
 monitoring during, 120–121
 percutaneous gastrostomy, 130–131
 positioning for, 121

respiratory effects of, 121
 timing of, 119–120
enoxaparin, for liver disease, 204
esomeprazole, for GERD, 5
esophageal varices, 168, 173
esophagogastroduodenoscopy. *See* endoscopy

famotidine, for GERD, 4, 6
fatty liver of pregnancy, 187, 200–202
fenofibrate, for pancreatitis disease, 158
fentanyl
 for endoscopy, 126
 for pancreatitis, 155
 preoperative, 140
fertility
 in inflammatory bowel disease, 92
 in liver disease, 167
flumazenil, for endoscopy, 124, 128
FODMAP diet, for irritable bowel syndrome, 82
Food and Drug Administration, medication classification of, 211–215
furosemide, for liver disease, 169

gallstones, 48–49, 141–145, 162–164
 pancreatitis in, 159–160
gastric bypass, pregnancy with, 31–37
 complications in, 33–34
 management of, 35–36
 nutritional issues in, 34–35
 pathophysiology of, 32–33
 statistics on, 31–32
gastroesophageal reflux disease, 1–11, 47
 evaluation of, 2–3
 pathophysiology of, 2
 presentation of, 2–3
 treatment of, 3–9
  agents for, 3–7
  selection of, 7–8
genetic factors, in inflammatory bowel disease, 92–93
GERD. *See* gastroesophageal reflux disease
gestational diabetes, gastric bypass and, 35
ginger, for nausea and vomiting, 22, 29
glucagon, for endoscopy, 128–129

heartburn, in GERD, 1–2
Helicobacter pylori infections, in nausea and vomiting, 15
HELLP syndrome, 187, 198–200
hematoma, liver, 200
hemorrhoids, 68–71, 147–148
heparin, for liver disease, 204

hepatic vein thrombosis, 192
hepatitis
    autoimmune, 177, 193
    nonalcoholic steatohepatitis, 179
hepatitis A, 186, 189, 204
hepatitis B, 204
    acute, 186, 190
    chronic, 174–175
hepatitis C, 175–176
hepatitis E, 186, 191
histamine H2-receptor antagonists, for GERD, 4, 6
hormones, in nausea and vomiting, 14–15
human chorionic gonadotropin, in nausea and vomiting, 14
hydralazine, for liver disease, 205
hydrocortisone
    for constipation, 67
    for hemorrhoids, 70
hydromorphone, for pancreatitis, 155
hydroxyzine
    for liver disease, 171, 178
    for nausea and vomiting, 27
hyoscyamine, for diarrhea, 83, 87
hyperemesis gravidarum, 16, 187, 194–195
hyperparathyroidism, pancreatitis in, 161
hypertension
    portal, 168, 173–174
    in pre-eclampsia, 198–200
hypoxia, in endoscopy, 121

imipenem, for pancreatitis, 156
immunoglobulin, for hepatitis B, 175, 204
immunomodulators, in inflammatory bowel disease, 98
infections
    abdominal pain in, 54–56
    respiratory, 54–55
    urinary tract, 55
inflammatory bowel disease, 45–46, 91–115
    breastfeeding in, 95–96, 100–104
    complications of, 104–105
    effects on pregnancy, 93–94
    endoscopic procedures for, 106–107
    epidemiology of, 91
    fertility in, 92
    inheritance of, 92–93
    laboratory studies in, 105
    mode of delivery in, 110
    nutrition in, 108–109
    pregnancy effects on, 94–95
    radiologic studies in, 105–106

treatment of
    biologic therapy, 102–104
    surgical, 107–108
infliximab, for inflammatory bowel disease, 98, 102–103
inheritance, of inflammatory bowel disease, 92–93
interferons, for liver disease, 170
intestinal obstruction, surgery for, 145–146
intrahepatic cholestasis of pregnancy, 187, 195–197
irritable bowel syndrome, 48, 75–89
    constipation in, 80, 83, 86
    criteria for, 75
    diagnosis of, 78–79
    diarrhea in, 80–81, 83–84, 87
    factors associated with, 77–78
    pain in, 82, 84–85, 87–88
    pathophysiology of, 78
    symptoms of, 76–77
    treatment of, 82–88
    work-up of, 80–82

Kaopectate, for diarrhea, 83, 87
kidney
    infections of, 55
    stones in, 50–51

labetalol, for liver disease, 205
lactation. *See* breastfeeding
lactulose
    for constipation, 65–66, 86
    for liver disease, 170
lamivudine, for liver disease, 170
lansoprazole, for GERD, 5, 6
laparoscopic adjustable gastric banding, 31–37
leiomyomas, uterine, 54
lidocaine, for endoscopy, 124, 129
lifestyle changes
    for GERD, 7
    for nausea and vomiting, 18
lithiasis, kidney, 50–51
liver
    adenomas of, 50
    disease of. *See* acute liver disease; chronic liver disease
    transplantation of, pregnancy after, 180
loperamide, for diarrhea, 83, 87
lubiprostone, for constipation, 67–68

magnesium citrate, for constipation, 66, 86

magnesium sulfate, for pre-eclampsia, 199

magnetic resonance cholangiopancreatography, 160

magnetic resonance imaging, for inflammatory bowel disease, 105–106

meclizine, for nausea and vomiting, 27

medications
  for biliary disease, 154–158
  classification of, during pregnancy, 211–215
  for constipation, 65–68
  for endoscopy, 122–129
  fetal risk summary for, 212–213
  for GERD, 9
  inadvertent exposure to, 213
  for inflammatory bowel disease, 96–102
  for irritable bowel syndrome, 82–88
  for liver disease, 169–172, 177–179, 192, 194–195, 197–200, 204–205
  liver injury due to, 186, 193–194
  for nausea and vomiting, 18–22, 27–29
  for pancreatitis, 154–158
  preoperative, 140
  prescribing decisions for, 213

meperidine
  for endoscopy, 122–123, 125
  for pancreatitis, 155
  preoperative, 140

6-mercaptopurine, for inflammatory bowel disease, 101–102

meropenem, for pancreatitis, 156

mesalamine, for inflammatory bowel disease, 97

methotrexate, for inflammatory bowel disease, 98

methylcellulose, for constipation, 65, 67

methylprednisolone, for nausea and vomiting, 21, 29

metoclopramide
  for GERD, 5, 7
  for nausea and vomiting, 20, 28

metronidazole
  for inflammatory bowel disease, 97, 99–100
  preoperative, 140

midazolam
  for endoscopy, 124, 127
  for pancreatitis, 157

mineral oil, for constipation, 66–67, 86

morphine
  for endoscopy, 123, 126
  for pancreatitis, 155
  preoperative, 140

motility, gastrointestinal, in nausea and vomiting, 15

mucosal protectants, for GERD, 4

Murphy's sign, in cholecystitis, 49

mycophenolate, for liver disease, 172, 180

naloxone, for endoscopy, 124, 127–128

natalizumab, for inflammatory bowel disease, 99, 104

nausea and vomiting, 13–29
  differential diagnosis of, 16–17
  epidemiology of, 14
  fetal protective nature of, 15–16
  nutritional considerations in, 23
  pathophysiology of, 14–16
  severe (hyperemesis gravidarum), 16
  testing for, 17
  treatment of, 18–22, 27–29

nephrolithiasis, 50–51

neuromodulators, for nausea and vomiting, 22

nifedipine, for liver disease, 205

nizatidine, for GERD, 4, 6

nonalcoholic steatohepatitis, 179

nutrition
  for gastric bypass, 34–35
  for inflammatory bowel disease, 108–109
  for nausea and vomiting, 23

obesity, gastric bypass for, 31–37

octreotide, for liver disease, 169

olsalazine, for inflammatory bowel disease, 97

omega-3 fatty acids, for pancreatitis, 157, 161

omeprazole, for GERD, 5

ondansetron, for nausea and vomiting, 21, 28

ovary
  masses in, 53
  torsion of, 53

oxygen supplementation, in endoscopy, 121

pain, abdominal. *See* abdominal pain

pancreatitis, 49–50, 153–162
  biliary, 159–160
  causes of, 159–161
  diagnosis of, 154

epidemiology of, 153
evaluation of, 159
outcomes of, 161–162
symptoms of, 154
treatment of, 154–158
pantoprazole, for GERD, 5
paroxetine, for irritable bowel syndrome, 88
pelvic inflammatory disease, 56
peptic ulcer disease, 46–47
piperacillin/tazobactam
  for pancreatitis, 156
  preoperative, 140
pneumonia, 54–55
polyethylene glycol
  for bowel preparation, 121, 125
  for constipation, 65–67, 86
portal hypertension, 168, 173–174
positioning, for endoscopy, 121
prednisone, for liver disease, 180
pre-eclampsia, 187, 198–200
primary biliary cirrhosis, 178
prochlorperazine, for nausea and vomiting, 20, 28
promethazine, for nausea and vomiting, 20, 27
promotility agents, for GERD, 5
propofol
  for endoscopy, 123, 126–127
  for pancreatitis, 157
propranolol, for liver disease, 169
proteinuria, in pre-eclampsia, 198–200
proton pump inhibitors
  for GERD, 5–6
  for nausea and vomiting, 21
pruritus, in intrahepatic cholestasis of pregnancy, 195–197
psychological counseling, for irritable bowel syndrome, 85
psyllium, for constipation, 65–66
pulmonary venous thromboembolism, 51–52
pyelonephritis, 55
pyrosis, in GERD, 1–2

rabeprazole, for GERD, 5
ranitidine, for GERD, 4, 6
reflux, gastroesophageal. *See* gastroesophageal reflux disease
respiratory considerations, in endoscopy, 121
ribavirin, for liver disease, 170
rifaximin, for liver disease, 170
Roux-en-Y gastric bypass, 31–37

sedation, for endoscopy, 122–127
seizures, in eclampsia, 198
senna, for constipation, 65–67, 86
serotonin antagonists
  for irritable bowel syndrome, 84–85, 88
  for nausea and vomiting, 21
sigmoidoscopy. *See* endoscopy
simethicone, for endoscopy, 125, 128
sirolimus, for liver disease, 180
sitz bath, for hemorrhoids, 70
small intestine, obstruction of, 44–45, 145–146
sodium bicarbonate, for GERD, 4
sodium phosphate
  for bowel preparation, 121
  for constipation, 66, 86
spironolactone, for liver disease, 169
splenic artery, aneurysm of, 53
steatohepatitis, nonalcoholic, 179
stones
  gallbladder, 48–49, 141–145, 159–160, 162–164
  kidney, 50–51
sucralfate, for GERD, 4, 7
sulfasalazine, for inflammatory bowel disease, 97
suppositories, for hemorrhoids, 70
surgery, 133–152
  for acute abdomen, 134
  for acute problems, 135–141
  bariatric. *See* gastric bypass
  for colorectal cancer, 148–149
  for hemorrhoids, 147–148
  for inflammatory bowel disease, 107–108
  initial management for, 134
  for intestinal obstruction, 145–147
  preoperative medications for, 140
  for urgent problems, 141–145

tacrolimus, for liver disease, 172, 180
tegaserol, for constipation, 68
thalidomide, for inflammatory bowel disease, 98
thromboembolism, pulmonary venous, 51–52
thrombosis, in Budd-Chiari syndrome, 186, 192–193
torsion, ovarian, 53
transplantation, liver, pregnancy after, 180
trauma, surgery for, 135–136
trientine, for liver disease, 172, 178
triglyceride-induced pancreatitis, 161
tube, cholecystostomy, `45

Turnbull-Blowhole colostomy, for inflammatory bowel disease, 107

ulcerative colitis. *See* inflammatory bowel disease
upper endoscopy. *See* endoscopy
urinary tract, infections of, 55
ursodeoxycholic acid, for liver disease, 171, 178, 197, 205
uterus, leiomyomas of, 54

vaccines, for viral hepatitis, 204
varices, esophageal, 168, 173
venography, for Budd-Chiari syndrome, 192

venous thromboembolism, pulmonary, 51–52
vitamin supplements
    for gastric bypass, 35
    for inflammatory bowel disease, 109
    for liver disease, 204–205
    for nausea and vomiting, 19, 27
vomiting. *See* nausea and vomiting

warfarin, for liver disease, 204
weight loss, gastric bypass for, 31–37
Wilson's disease, 178–179

zinc sulfate, for liver disease, 172, 178–179

Printed in the United States
by Baker & Taylor Publisher Services